What's Eating You?

A Food Reference Manual

(Revised)

Rebekah S. Mead

What's Eating You?
A Food Reference Manual
(Revised)

ISBN 978-10-762020-86
Copyright 2019

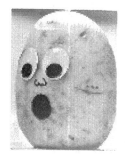

Cover created by Ron Fortin

This book is available through Amazon.com and Amazon Kindle

Rebekah@whatseatingyou.info

Rebekah S. Mead

Acknowledgments

First and foremost, thank you, John Briggs, for bringing me back to my roots and helping me re-establish my organic diet and garden. If not for you, I would not have had this time to research and write my first book.

Likewise, I much appreciate Kate Branton for her belief in me and ongoing encouragement. We have shared great conversations about our healthcare system, and the impact industrial food has had on health in America. Her professional healthcare knowledge aroused my desire to delve into evidence-based research, and as a cherished friend, together, we wonder why this information isn't common knowledge?

I have much gratitude for the painting Ron Fortin painted for the cover of my book.

Also, I have tremendous respect for all of the members of my writing group, the Port Orange Scribes of the Florida Writing Association. They encouraged me to keep writing and provided much-needed advice.

My acknowledgments wouldn't be complete without mentioning the Institute for Responsible Technology (IRT). This organization kindled my interest in food safety and disease prevention when I attended an Energy Fest in Kempton, Pa., in 2004. The keynote speaker was Jeffery Smith Ph.D., author of Seeds of Deception and founder of the IRT. His lecture made me aware of how food in America was and continues to be covertly altered and changed in many ways without adequate regulations or premarket testing before selling to consumers. His organization opened my eyes to the fact that the food industry is self-regulated. Their food labels are not required to disclose relevant information that could prevent health problems in some people. As a nurse, I realized how little I knew about these changes. Since then, I have delved into evidence-based research so to understand how food additives and genetically engineered foods affect our health and healthcare system in the same way they are intended to harm and repel pests.

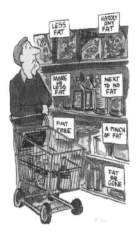

Preface

The American diet has changed immensely ever since the deregulation of genetically altered plants and animals and its use in our food. Legislation of the 1990s brought about genetically engineered crops and farmed animals with industrial genes that repel or kill any pests that attempt to consume them. When put into our food, many of these crops have the same effect on our health as it was intended to have on the pests.

As a nurse, I witnessed the increase in chronic illnesses and the rise in new ailments over this last generation. When patients were prescribed medication, I used a drug reference manual to identify the risks and side-effects and used that information to educate those I cared for. But, no such reference manual is available for all the products of biotechnological additives in our food. Therefore, I decided to create a series of books for public use. How the food we eat today becomes our immune system and cholesterol of tomorrow should be common knowledge. Understanding how specific food additives affect our health is necessary to prevent preventable illnesses.

This book explains the process of how consumed food become life-sustaining elements. Each section describes how the food put into our mouth today breaks-down into nutrients that your body will use to make enzymes, hormones, cholesterol, and many other necessary compounds needed to function correctly. It is intended to be the first of a series that consumers can use to identify which food additives may be causing their problems in their health.

There are *Key Points* at the end of each chapter for anyone who prefers a brief overview. The last section is the beginning of my list of chemicals, their risks, and their side-effects.

Whichever order is most natural to understand is the best order to read it in. I encourage everyone to look up the references for additional insights. The goal is to raise awareness; to make consumers aware:

➤ Of the changes made to food in the last twenty-five years.

➤ What chemicals and pesticides you are eating.

➤ Food additives and Products of Biotechnology (POB's) have side effects, just like medications do. Some may even change the effectiveness of your prescribed medications.

➤ Ingredients that are impossible to pronounce are chemicals that should be investigated before consuming to be sure they are not making you sick.

➤ What is the *maximum safe limit* of each additive to consume daily?

➤ Food determined to be *Generally Recognized as Safe* (GRAS) is not monitored or regulated by the FDA or USDA. They are thought to be generally safe when consumed in moderate amounts by healthy people.

➤ Which additives cause or increase your symptoms?

➤ Some food-additives are intended to increase your appetite and food cravings? These foods can be making you obese, lazy, agitated, and sick?

Diseases caused by food are preventable illnesses. By eliminating disease-causing food from our diet, we can reduce our nation's overall healthcare costs by as much as 75%. That is a $3 trillion annual savings all Americans can strive for together. As a country, we can reduce the cost of health care by preventing preventable illnesses caused by the food we eat.

Rebekah S. Mead

Table of Contents

Rebekah S. Mead

Introduction

"The most important practical lesson that can be given to nurses is to teach them what to observe - how to observe - what symptoms indicate improvement - what to reverse - which are of importance - which are of none - which are the evidence of neglect - and of what kind of neglect."   – Florence Nightingale

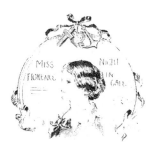

Do you know what to avoid before having a severe reaction? Or do, would you know if specific ingredients are causing long term effects on your health?

One of the main problems with choosing healthy foods is that lawmakers throughout the last twenty-five years have made it legal to make genetic alterations to our foods and the labeling of scientifically cultivated food voluntary. Since 1994, food producers who have concerns that American consumers will not buy their product if it is known to be potentially harmful to our health, have laws that protect their right not to mention any warning on their labels. This generation of government officials has passed laws that make food labeling voluntary.

Most likely you have consumed Genetically Modified Organisms (GMO) today and every day for the past two decades, because of more than 75% of all foods sold in America since 1996 contain scientifically made ingredients using some form of biotechnology. In this book, I refer to these scientifically-engineered foods as, Products of Biotechnology (POB).

The food industry in the USA is not required to disclose how their food-products are cultivated. Therefore, you may not be aware that some of the foods you consume may be causing your health problems, if you have any, (Hauck, 2014), (Spear, 2015).

Growing numbers of food products are now made using Genetically Modified Organisms (GMO) and Genetically Engineered (GE) ingredients. In 1996, almost no crops in the United States used genetic engineering. The USDA estimates that today, over 80% of American grown soybeans and corn are GMO or GE. Animal-based GMO foods are also increasing. For example, USDA has approved the sale of GE salmon. Studies estimate that over 75% of processed foods sold in grocery stores contain GMO ingredients. To date, there is no federal requirement to label GE or GMO foods. Multiple consumer movements have been organized in the United States to join the other countries around the world that require labeling of foods that contain GMO or GE ingredients, (Rose, http://lawatlas.org/datasets/gmo-al, 2016).

The first GMO crop to be sold in the USA was the Flavr-Savr tomato. Unbeknownst to the average consumer and healthcare providers, in 1996, these GMO tomatoes were unassumingly placed amongst the organic tomatoes in the produce aisle. They looked like ordinary tomatoes because organic tomatoes were used to create them, but that is where their similarity ended. Aside from their lack of flavor, those tomatoes contained genes from seafood, E-coli, and the antibiotic Kanamycin. If you were allergic to shellfish or had an autoimmune deficiency, you may have experienced a reaction without knowing the cause. There was no indication of any sort on the label to warn anyone who may react to these hidden genes. And, medical professionals were not made aware of any potential health risks. Therefore, patients who reacted to those GMO tomatoes were diagnosed with symptoms of unknown origin. Those who suffered severe allergic reactions were not instructed to avoid Flavr Savr tomatoes.

Today, some infant formulas contain additives that have no nutrient value and can even cause health problems. Ingredients may come from trans-genetic cows that share human genes that make them produce human milk, (Yang B, 2011), (Stevenson, H., 2014). The Weston A. Price Foundation attributes the rise in violence by young men against each other during this past generation to pesticide residue, genetically altered food, and additives that act like medications in our food when broken down in our digestive system.

According to the Weston Price Foundation, "In the 1990s, a new form of deadly violence raised its head in America. There was an escalating pattern of chilling destruction aimed at students and carried out by students, violence that increases every year. From the 1999 Columbine shootings in Colorado to the recent shootings, Americans are desperately searching for answers"(Price 2008).

The social anxiety and aggression seen in the USA today are in sharp contrast with Dr. Weston Price's descriptions of other more fun-loving, well-nourished indigenous cultures. From smiling, joyful South Sea Islanders to highly spiritual Gaelic fisherfolk to Swiss villagers enjoying their peaceful lives (Price, 2008). Likewise, Dr. Francis Pettniger described friendly, harmonious behavior among well-nourished cats. Pettinger's study revealed how both cats and humans degenerated into disharmonious behavior patterns with the change to foods that were devitalized by heat and processing (Price, 2008).

"Modern commentators are blind to the solution, a solution that is in plain sight: clearly defining good nutrition and putting it back into the mouths of our children, starting before they are conceived... because food is information and that information directly affects the emotions, the nervous system, the brain, and behavior" (Onusic, 2013).

The lack of research before the sale of such products is a severe threat to the health of all life forms. The notion of altering nature for the betterment of humankind assumes that the rest of nature has no value and is sacrificed through unlimited and unmonitored POB research and food production.

I remember sitting on my breezeway with my sister-in-law while our children played in the yard. We were concerned about the prospect of aspartame added to food and beverages. Back then, everything we read about aspartame indicated that it could alter brain-wave patterns and cause harm to the nervous system. Aspartame can also stimulate our appetite, making us crave more of that food. I recall reading this damage was reversible in adults who stopped consuming it, but irreversible in teens and children. Being pregnant at the time, I was concerned about research claiming that by drinking aspartame while pregnant, it could cause neurological damage and learning disabilities in the fetus and increase the risk for postpartum depression. We were both upset when the media announced aspartame was GRAS added to most diet beverages and foods. Upon its approval by the FDA, the best we could do as consumers were to not foods with this additive.

13

To all Americans, my advice is: What we buy is a vote for those products, and what we refuse to buy is also a vote to get it off our supermarket shelves.

For more than two decades, food engineers and scientists have used enormous amounts of organic resources to cultivate their man-made products. Their products are used in the food they produce and for further laboratory experimentation. All the while, they are performing somewhat of an ethnic cleansing of Mother Nature. Their goal is to control all forms of organic life by mixing genes and creating chemicals that repel and kill the environment.

The food producers own the technology to make these foods and implement patents that prevent competition. When human DNA added to that of an ordinary cow, it becomes a company commodity.

Imagine if all cows were exterminated or replaced with cows containing human genes: GMO soy that bleeds imitation blood would replace naturally-nutritious hamburgers; milk, butter, cheese, ice cream, and all other dairy products would contain patented imitation dairy products made by some company that would own all of the rights to those genes and seeds. Much like pharmaceuticals today, the price and availability of food would depend on the whims of the food industry.

The environment in which we live today affects the food and beverages we consume. The cultivation of plants and animals affects not only our land, water, and air, but also that of wildlife. While individuals may choose what types of food they eat, their options are limited to what is available in their environment, e.g., stores, restaurants, schools, and worksites (CDC, 2009), (NEL, 2012).

Prior to 1994, food portions were as much as 3/4th less than they are today, and the general population in the USA was physically healthier (Scinta, 2016). Food and agriculture have changed a lot in just two and a half decades, whereas most consumers, including medical professionals, are still not fully aware of its effects on our health and our economy. Throughout my diverse career as a nurse, I have never witnessed medical professionals' rule-out food additives and chemicals as a cause for symptoms. When I mentioned GMO and POB foods to my colleagues, they look at me like I have two heads!

Since the onset of deregulated POB foods, there has been a tremendous amount of international research performed that concludes eating strictly organic (real natural food) satisfies hunger quicker while meeting more nutritional needs. People who purely consume unaltered real food are satisfied with up to three-fourths less food and have less incidence of diseases and degenerative disorders, which are said to be *preventable chronic illnesses*.

In 2017, the Center for Diseases Control and Prevention (CDC) released a report stating, "90% of our nations $3.5 trillion in annual medical care expenditure was spent on people with chronic medical conditions," (CDC, 2017), (Buttorff C, Multiple chronic conditions in the United States, 2017), (Center for Medicare & Medicaid Services, 2017). That equals $3.15 trillion spent on preventable chronic illnesses in the USA every year.

To me, this indicates that Americans can reduce our medical costs by $3.15 trillion by merely eating only nutritious foods known not to cause harm, be physically active and get the right amount of sleep every day. These are lifestyle choices that support a long productive life with no chronic illnesses. Relying on elected officials and medical professionals will not cut it. Only we the people can take control of our health to turn this country around.

Anyone who claims they cannot afford the high price of organic foods is not aware that buying and consuming as much as one-fourth the quantity of POB foods will reduce both their food bills and health care expenses by up to 75%, which are huge savings. Many consumers don't shop around. Competitors of organic foods may offer a store incentive to charge higher prices for their comparable organic foods.

I recently had such an experience when my friend purchased two dozen cage-free, organically certified eggs and a gallon of organic milk for $18.99. It was a supermarket known for lower prices, but he spent more than double what I paid for the same brands at another store known for having organic foods at lower prices. I paid $2.99 per dozen eggs and $4.99 for a gallon of the brand of milk, both products were the same brands with the same expiration dates, but I paid a total of $10.97. Buyer beware.

What I now know is when I create homemade meals and baked-goodies using 100% organic ingredients, the taste, and texture are wonderful, but even more rewarding is that I feel fuller faster, I eat less and spend less on food while having more energy to do the things I enjoy.

If your health and quality of life aren't incentive enough to make necessary lifestyle changes, consider the environment and wildlife. While unwittingly exposed to these products, through cultivation and consumption, the demand and cost of medical care have increased dramatically. Domestic and wildlife have also been affected in ways that harm all life. According to the Canadian Council on Animal Care, trans-genetic animals are organic plants, animals, and bacteria that have been scientifically altered by means such as the consumption of GMO foods, cloning life, or genetically changing the DNA. Animals that have undergone "induced mutations" require special care related to the stability of induced traits that are not natural (Ormandy,

15

2011). Human diseases that did not affect pets in the past are now causing chronic human-ailments in our pets, which are requiring more expensive veterinary care.

The ethical issues raised by human-animal transgenesis, human rights, and religious activists raise the question of how much DNA it takes to make other animals human? We have an elected official whose 0.09% native Indian DNA made her eligible to go to a prestigious college as their first female of color; does this mean that a cow that originally has sixty DNA chromosomes and then has three strands replaced with human DNA is now 5% human?

How does this affect the meat and dairy products derived from these animals? What percentage of our natural resources are being used to raise these commodities? Considering that less than 30% will turn out as intended, this is a big waste of natural resources, because, those that do not contain the desired traits as expected by the scientists get euthanized. How does their disposal affect the environment and our economy? (Tonti-Filippini, 2001).

Most people, including healthcare professionals (doctors, nurses, registered dieticians, and veterinarians), know very little about the effects that unnatural foods have on humans and other animals in the environment. Mental and physical illnesses and degenerative changes had significantly increased since the year 2000 when President Clinton and Prime Minister Tony Blair announced, "Today, we are learning the language in which God created life. With this profound new knowledge, humankind is on the verge of gaining immense, new power to heal." (Clinton, 2000).

This should have triggered urgent environmental and scientific monitoring within this country, but it hasn't. Instead, new foods are created and sold every year without our knowledge. Any adverse effects caused by newly invented foods go undetected until enough people are harmed to raise a concern about the product's safety. In the meantime, American medical professionals are continuously treating new disorders caused by these unregulated products.

In communities with a high incidence of heart disease, cancer, autoimmunity disorders, degenerative disease, and mental illness that includes violence, are our public health officials performing adequate health-risk analyses on the environment? Are our tax dollars being used to implement changes that mitigate the damage POB foods cause to each community? According to research, the nation's receiving foreign aid in the form of POB foods is now experiencing an increase is diabetes, heart disease, obesity, cancer, and degenerative disorders in addition to their original malnutrition?

One study indicates that the global rise in diabetes requires so much additional insulin that will be in short-supply by 2030 (Lapidus, 2018).

While scientists work hard to change our food, we must ask ourselves truthfully, is it helping the planet more than it is harming it. "Economic development and the evolution of the food industry not only help to meet the human needs for food but also cause worldwide health problems. Due to the imbalance of economic development and the difference in dietary habits, the population in China is faced with the problem of excessive food intake, obesity, and the possible deficiency of some nutrients. In the past few decades, the food industry has profoundly affected people's intake patterns of nutrients such as energy, fat, salt, and added sugar, as well as changed the nutritional structure of food and the risk of exposure to harmful substances. Food contaminations caused by pathogenic microorganisms, pesticides, and heavy metals are serious concerns. The dietary guidelines for Chinese residents provide basic principles for guiding the dietary behaviors of the public, but their implementation is hampered by people's lack of understanding of food and nutrition, traditional dietary habits, media misinformation, and other factors. How to provide healthy and safe food for people is an important issue at present. This paper discusses some basic concepts of a healthy diet, how to promote healthy eating habits through education, how to preserve and process food to maintain nutrition, how to control food safety hazards, and other dietary related approaches that can promote health," (Yang, 2019).

Interestingly, a Physicians' Drug Reference manual (PDR) is updated every year for medical professionals to understand the intent, potential adverse interactions, and side-effects of approved medications. But, in spite of the massive amount of international Evidence-Based Research (EBR) proving the effects of GMO and POB food additives, there is no standardized general Food Reference Manual (FRM) to help consumers make informed decisions about their health.

Like why?

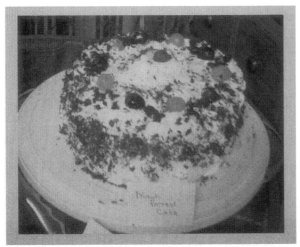

My Black Forest Cake after switching to 100% heavy cream with no additives, high gluten organic flour, and eggs from cage-free, organically fed chickens

Have you noticed that homemade snacks and meals do not turn out the way they used to? Have you tried to replicate recipes made by your mom thirty years ago, but they don't taste the same, nor do they have the succulent texture you remember?

Have you tried cooking an old traditional family recipe lately? Factory farmed egg whites are too watery to whip into fluffy mounds of meringue. Processed flour is a light powdery filler that neither thickens gravy or rises in baked goods, and heavy whipping cream does not whip into thick fluffy whipped cream. These three primary products lack texture and taste, not to mention their nutritional values.

For over a decade, I struggled to make my old recipes look and taste like they used to. I gave up gardening long ago because the seeds I bought no longer produced the quality or quantity of crops I desired. I was so desperate for a flourishing garden that bought soil infused with chemical promising wonderous results, but nothing compared to my garden back when I lived on the farm where I grew up.

It wasn't until I started investigating the cause that I realized how much genetically engineered plants and animals had affected the food in America. The change from organic to POB was somewhat slow enough to be subtle, making Americans unaware of its impact on our mental and physical health.

I expressed my frustration to family, friends, and any acquaintances willing to listen to my complaints about how my old favorite recipes never turn out the way they used to. Most of these people seemed like they just had an epiphany, claiming they too could not make homemade meals that are appealing and satisfying.

Family dinners used to be a popular weekly event, if not more frequent. Making homemade meals from my garden-fresh crops and meat grown by local farmers was half the joy of preparing these meals. But as ingredients changed, making tasty meals that were also nutritious became more difficult, whereas serving premade processed meals grew tiresome. Often at least one food did not agree with someone, and most complained of being bloated and gassy after meals. These gatherings grew fewer and fewer until they ended.

When I finally switched to organic ingredients, the taste and texture of my old recipes returned. I was relieved to realize I had not lost my flair for cooking. The culprit was the quality of food and food additives sold in supermarkets across the country.

My recollection of a time before lawmakers deregulated GMO and POB foods were of a time when I was still living on my family's farm within a large farming community. As a nurse, I commuted over an hour in either direction into the inner cities to work. Back home on the farm, my mom and children continued to eat natural foods grown on our farm, but when I was working, my eating habits changed dramatically. I worked twelve and sixteen-hour shifts with no meal breaks. I usually ordered something from a local delivery place or skipped meals altogether. My food sat on the nurse's station, where I picked at it when I had a few moments here and there. My sleep habits also became erratic; I often went days without sleep.

I began to gain weight. My health suffered as did my vitality. I often felt pain on my right side after meals. Other times I broke out in hives, which had not happened during my youth. I even went through phases when I felt painfully bloated and had to rush to the bathroom with explosive diarrhea, none of which I experienced previously during my life on the farm and before becoming a registered nurse. All the while, my mom and son remained thin, even though their appetites were hearty. After a full day of activities and dinner, they sat together on the couch, passing a jar of creamy peanut butter back-and-forth as each dipped their miniature chocolate candy bars into the real peanut butter. Meanwhile, I ate more and more fat-free foods and grew more and more frustrated with my weight.

I will never forget this one day; I was exhausted from multiple long shifts back to back.

We had finished eating a healthy dinner hours ago when I snuggled into my favorite chair across from the couch where mom and Rob sat to snack on their usual treats. I was holding a hand-full of tasteless fat-free cookies. I can still hear mom's soft voice from across the room, saying, "Ya, know Beck, I bet all that fat-free food you eat is what's making you fat!"

As much as I adored everything about my mom ever since I was a child and every memory of her still brings me great joy, at that moment in my life, I was so outraged that I wanted to smack the jar of creamy, delightful--smelling peanut-butter out of her hand. Instead, I debated the benefits of eating fat-free food, and then consumed the entire package of cookies, all 12 servings, because it did not satisfy my appetite. In fact, they made me hungrier.

The way the two of them could eat anything, french-fries made in bacon fat, butter slather on toast anything, and never gained an ounce was the way I used to be. And I was frustrated.

Coincidently, that was the time when fat-free foods hit the marketplace and advertised heavily as healthy. I was a professional registered Intensive Care Unit (ICU) nurse at that time, yet my healthcare colleagues nor I discussed the potential risks of all the changes made to food, and we certainly didn't correlate its side-effects to the increase in chronic illnesses. There was no continuing education training offered to warn us about the adverse side-effects, which is unusual; continuing education is a nursing requirement to keep us informed and updated about any trends that impact health. There was no evidence-based-research to read on our own because none was performed before releasing these scientific experiments into the American food supply.

In intensive care units, patients admitted with heart attacks received no-fat diets, and then their symptoms usually got worse. Before long, the medical providers realized healthy fat is needed to absorb vital fat-soluble vitamins. Thereby a fat-free diet was causing malnutrition in those who were already struggling with heart disease. Within a few years, this protocol changed to a low-fat diet.

So many years have passed since that day. Whereas the evolution of foods sold to American consumers has been constant, its impact on my life has been more of a gradual learning curve. What I've discovered is:

☺ My favorite old recipes require organic ingredients to maintain their flavor, nutrient value, and texture. Non-organic ingredients cause unpredictable results. Baked goods flop, soupy omelets burn quickly, heavy cream diluted with water, and carrageenan will not whisk into fluffy whipped cream, and unnatural ingredients have unnatural tastes.

☺   In 2013, when meat started making me nauseous and sick, I unconsciously became a pescatarian. My health problems disappeared when I switched to organic foods. After meals, I used to feel painfully bloated with gallbladder pain and generalized irritable bowel syndrome. I experienced new allergies to processed foods - my tongue swelled, tingled, and sometimes I had difficulty breathing. Often my mouth and lips were so numb that I couldn't taste what I was eating. Since I cut out food and additives that make me sick, all my symptoms have disappeared, naturally.

☺   When I switched to organic seeds in organic soil, my garden began to flourish again.

Throughout my life, I've met many people experiencing the same health problems that I had. As a nurse, I was able to share my experiences in such a way as to help others make better lifestyle choices. I very much agree with Florence Nightingale, who once said, "If a patient is sick after taking food, it is not the fault of the disease. Fresh air, fresh food, and exercise are needed."

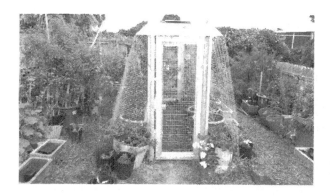

In recent years, I have come to appreciate nature, our environment, and its history much more than ever before. In 1862, Abraham Lincoln created "The Peoples Department," which later became the United States Department of Agriculture (USDA). This department was first created to advance farming while protecting the environment as America moved into the industrial age. At that time, 98% of all Americans were farmers to some degree. Whether they had a small farm to produce only enough food for their family or a more substantial farmer who sold their crops, less than 2% of Americans did not work the soil, natural plant seeds, milk their cows and collect eggs. Every community had a butcher who either slaughtered their farmed animals or sold meats grown locally.

Growing up on a farm in the 1960s and 1970s, I remember parents forcing their children to eat, because "there are starving children in Ethiopia." I was no different. I worked then played outside from dawn to dusk and had little interest in food until I was old enough to grow my small garden. It was only later when I first grew radishes and then graduated to bigger crops that I began to enjoy anything and everything that came from my labor.

I remember friends saying, "there nothing like a Jersey tomato. And they were right! I could make a meal on the tender skin and sweet flesh of any tomatoes grown in the clay soil that was natural to the area. What amazed me was the seeds I saved from each plant I grew always germinated into another generation of crops. A tiny tomato seed could grow six feet tall and produce two or more dozen sweet juicy tomatoes.

Natural food was just a part of life; the nearest grocery store was about an hour away, so my family processed much of our food. Fresh cream skimmed off the unpasteurized milk that was agitated by hand in an old wood-churn into butter. Free-range chickens produced fresh eggs each day, meat kept in a freezer, and garden vegetables were canned or frozen for the winter months. We had a large apple orchard on our farm that was not used by us, but we had more than enough fresh apples to eat and make dumplings and pies.

Life was full of adventure, both good and bad. Before I was old enough to get a job, I shoveled manure in barns for local farmers and babysat occasionally. Other kids in the neighborhood mowed lawns and raked leaves. The exercise was free, with all calories burned by the time bedtime rolled around. Sleep came easy. I was usually asleep before my head hit the pillow. A virtue I am still blessed to have still.

On occasions when anyone got injured, our local doctor saw us any time of the day or night. He treated our injuries, and soon we felt better. I can't remember a time that my mom or dad had to wait in a sitting-room. Before leaving Dr. Liby's office, my dad pulled out his wallet and paid him for a visit.

As of 2016, less than 2% of people in America are farmers. Farming accounts for about 1% percent of the U.S. Gross Domestic Product (GDP), whereas the US farmed food and fiber exports were $135.5 billion (American

Farm Bureau Federation, 2019). That same year, 2016, Americans spent 17% of the U.S GDP on medical care. National medical care reached $3.4 trillion (Baron, 2019), which is more than double what any other nation spends on all of their health care (OECD, 2018). According to the World Health Organization (WHO), the U.S. spends a higher portion of its gross domestic product on medical care than any other country but ranks only 37 out of 191 countries in quality of care and outcomes. The United Kingdom, which spends just six percent of GDP on health services, ranks 18th" (WHO, 2018).

Compared to half a century ago, children in America today cannot stop eating, their energy is low, and work is considered abusive. Obesity amongst children ages 6 to 19 has tripled between 1980 and 2004 (CDC, 2007) and then doubled again through 2014 (Dabrowska, 2014). In fact, one researcher at the academy of pediatrics medicine estimates 43% of all children in America have at least one chronic condition (Bethell, 2011). Allergies and obesity are major problems for children.

Peanut butter used to be a staple high in protein, but now because of cross-pollination with GMO grains such as soy, it is banned in many schools due to allergic reactions.

"Peanut allergy prevalence quadrupled from 0.4 percent in 1997 to more than 2 percent in 2010. It is now the leading cause of anaphylactic shock, the most severe form of allergy, due to food in the United States" (Porterfield, 2017).

"In 2007, approximately 3 million children under age 18 years (3.9%) were reported to have a food allergy. From 1997 to 2007, the prevalence of food allergies increased 18% among children under age 18 years. Children with food allergies are four times more likely to develop other conditions such as asthma and other allergies, compared with children without food allergies. From 2004 to 2006, there were approximately 9,500 hospital discharges per year with a diagnosis related to food allergy among children under age 18 years" (Branum, 2008).

Food allergy is a potentially serious immune response to eating specific foods or food additives. Eight types of food account for over 90% of allergic reactions in affected individuals: milk, eggs, peanuts, tree nuts, fish, shellfish, soy, and wheat. Reactions to these foods by an allergic person can range from a tingling sensation around the mouth and lips and hives to death, depending on the severity of the allergy. The mechanisms by which a person develops an allergy to specific foods are largely unknown (Branum, 2008).

Genetically Modified Organisms (GMO) "soy ingredients are in more than 60% of processed or packaged foods and nearly 100% of fast foods"

(Jennifer, 2013). Soy is even used to make hamburgers that bleed man-made blood (Rainer, 2018). Soy, in the form of vegetable-textured-protein, replaces meat in products such as stuffed clams and meat ravioli.

"People who are allergic to soy may also react to eggs, dairy, and fresh foods. Their symptoms are usually chalked up to multiple allergies, but the cause might well be soy residues from the soy-based chows fed to poultry, cows, sheep, and fish before consumption" (Daniels, 2012).

"In 2001, Biotechnology researchers from the Food Research and Development Laboratories of the Honen Corporation, of Shizuoka, Japan, described feeding hens a diet containing a high concentration of soy isoflavones and then measured the isoflavones in plasma and egg yolk. Over eighteen days, the strength of isoflavones peaked on the twelfth day with isoflavone levels in the egg yolk at 65.29 µg per 100 g. This value remained constant throughout the rest of the experiment" (Daniels, 2012).

In 2009, grad student Dante Miguel Marcial Vargas Galdos at Ohio State University completed a master's thesis entitled Quantification of Soy Isoflavones in Commercial Eggs and their Transfer from Poultry Feed into Eggs and Tissue. In this study, forty-eight laying hens were fed three types of chicken feed: a soy-free feed, a regular feed containing 25 percent soybean meal, and a special feed that packed 500 mg soy isoflavones per 100 grams.

Vargas Galdos' study successfully proved that the isoflavones in chicken feed transferred and accumulated into the hen eggs and tissues. Chickens fed the special-blend of chow with the extra 500 mg isoflavones per 100 grams laid eggs with yolks containing 1000 µg isoflavones per 100 grams. Chicken livers, kidneys, hearts and muscles contained 7162 µg per 100g, 3355 µg per 100g, 272 µg per 100g and 97 µg per 100g, respectively. He found no soy isoflavones in the eggs laid by hens fed soy-free Coco-feed obtained from Tropical Traditions. Although these chickens had grown up on the regular 25 percent soy protein feed, no trace of soy isoflavones remained in their eggs ten days after switching to the soy-free alternative. (Saitoh, Sato, Harada, & Takita, 2001).

"The obvious question is, why so many reactions, and why now? The main reason appears to be the increased number of allergenic proteins found in GMO soy. According to previous research and the Peanut Genome Initiative, it appears that in the genetic engineering of soy, a soy allergen is 41 percent identical to a known peanut allergen. This new allergen, now found in soy, is recognized by 44 percent of peanut-allergic individuals. Recent studies out of the University of London, support this research and highlight the role that GMO soy and soy formula play in the development of the peanut allergy. In the United States, 90 percent of soy contains these new proteins, chemicals, and allergens." (Daniels, 2012).

An even more curious question is, why are peanuts banned from some schools, but GMO soy is not?

In supermarkets, many mysterious ingredients and metaphors listed on food labels are quite often downright misleading. How our elected lawmakers regulate the food sold in America and specifically define "natural ingredients" is not always consistent with the one-hundred-and-thirty other nations that have since signed the Cartagena Act; an agreement not to cultivate or sell any food products until proven to cause no harm to humans or their environment. In fact, many POB and food additives are banned from use in food products in those nations for safety reasons, yet our regulatory agencies have approved their use by food producers. Hormone disrupting pesticides and other biocides leave residues on produce sold in markets that are known to have adverse effects on certain people. When most American consumers do not immediately experience adverse reactions upon consumption in the quantities recommended, our tax-funded Food and Drug Administration (FDA) categorizes those ingredients as Generally Recognized as Safe (GRAS) and therefore do not need to be monitored.

So, what happens when someone eats more than one portion or consumes many foods with the same risks? Worse yet, what if you fall into the minority category that does experience adverse side-effects? How do you and your medical provider know those ingredients are the culprit causing your symptoms?

You don't because, for the past twenty-five years, our legislators have made labeling GMO and POB foods voluntary. If the food industry feels consumers will not buy products containing unsafe ingredients, they have the legal right not to inform us. Any legislators who attempted to make labeling mandatory for the sake of protecting its citizens were met with strong opposition by the 114th congress that made it illegal for any state in the USA to mandate labeling GMO and POB foods, via their H.R. 1599 Act, (114 Congress , 2015), (Stevenson, 2014).

Many human, animal, and environmental activists call the H.R. 1599 Act, the "Monsanto Protection Act," or the "DARK act," which stands for "Denying Americans the Right to Know." Their concern is the lack of testing before selling products that may harm the environment and the refusal of our elected officials to sign the Cartagena Protocols.

The environment in which we live today affects the food and beverages we consume. How plants and animals are cultivated affects our land, water, and air, all of which affect our health. While individuals may choose the food they eat, their choices are limited to what is available in their environment, e.g., stores, restaurants, schools, and worksites (CDC, 2009), (NEL, 2012).

Since the onset of deregulated POB foods, there has been a tremendous amount of international evidence-based-research performed that is now available and concludes eating strictly organic (real natural food) satisfies hunger better while meeting all nutritional needs. People who purely consume unaltered real food are satisfied with up to three-fourths less food and have less incidence of diseases and degenerative disorders, which is also known as preventable chronic illnesses.

In 2017, our Center for Diseases Control and Prevention (CDC) released a report stating, "90% of our nations $3.5 trillion in annual medical care expenditure were spent on people with chronic medical conditions," (CDC, 2017), (Buttorff C, Multiple chronic conditions in the United States, 2017), (Center for Medicare & Medicaid Services, 2017). That equals $3.15 trillion spent on preventable chronic illnesses in the USA in just one year.

To me, this indicates that consumers can prevent $3.15 trillion in medical costs by merely eating only nutritious foods known not to cause harm, be physically active and get the right amount of sleep every day. These are lifestyle choices that support a long productive life with no chronic illnesses. We, the people, can take control of our health to turn this country around.

Those who claim they cannot afford the high price of organic foods are not aware that organic foods satisfy hunger quicker, resulting in eating as much as half the amount compared to POB foods. When you create homemade meals and treats made with naturally-organic ingredients, you can taste the difference while feeling fuller sooner. This can be a considerable saving in grocery and medical bills.

If your health and quality of life aren't incentive enough to make necessary lifestyle changes, consider the environment. When genes and other food elements, and chemicals are patented, food producers then have full control over prices and availability. Profits can cause producers to grow an imbalance of crops that do not meet the needs of consumers.

Most people, including healthcare professionals (doctors, nurses, registered dieticians, and veterinarians) know very little about the effects that unnatural foods have on humans, and other animals, in the environment. Mental and physical illness and degenerative changes have significantly increased since the late 1990s that should have triggered urgent environmental and scientific research within this country, but it hasn't. The curriculum of higher education for healthcare providers lack information about POB foods and their impact on health, and the environment is virtually ignored.

While unwittingly exposed to these products, through cultivation and consumption, the demand and cost of medical care have increased dramatically. Domestic and wildlife have also been affected in ways that harm all life. According to the Canadian Council on Animal Care, trans-genetic animals are created by scientifically altering naturally-organic animals. The transfer of foreign DNA from unrelated species is achieved through one of three methods: By the consumption of GMO foods, cloning life, or genetically changing the DNA of plants and animals. Animals that have undergone "induced mutations" require special care related to the stability of induced traits that are not natural (Ormandy, 2011). As a result, human diseases that did not affect pets in the past are now causing chronic human ailments in our pets, which requires more expensive veterinary care.

As for ethical issues of human-animal transgenesis, human right and religious activists raise the question of how much DNA makes an animal-human? We have an elected official whose 0.09% native Indian DNA made her eligible to go to a prestigious college as their first female of color; does this mean that when a cow that had sixty original DNA cow-chromosomes has three strands of DNA replaced with human DNA, is now 5% human? Does that cow now have human rights?

How does this affect the meat and dairy products derived from these animals? How does its manure affect the environment? With only 30% of transgenetic animals successfully turn out as intended by the scientists who create them, 70% of the natural resources used, were a waste. The 70% of transgenetic animals that do not contain the traits desired are then euthanized. Is this not an animal rights concern? And, how does their disposal affect the environment and our economy (Tonti-Filippini, 2001)?

In communities with a high incidence of heart disease, cancer, autoimmunity disorders, degenerative disease and mental illness that includes violence, are our public health officials performing adequate health-risk analyses on the environment and are our tax dollars being used to implement changes to prevent and reverse the damage POB foods cause to each community?

Interestingly, a Physicians' Drug Reference manual (PDR) is updated every year for medical professionals to understand the intent, potential adverse interactions and side-effects of approved medications, but with all of the international research available about the effects of GMO and POB food additives, no such database has been used to create a Food Reference Manual (FRM) to help consumers make informed decisions about their health.

The GE food industry asserts it is resolving world hunger. Where is the evidence-based-research proving that assertion? Most evidence-based research indicates there is a growing global epidemic of malnutrition compounded by obesity and diabetes. Making people fat and sick has not solved hunger.

According to research, those nation's receiving POB foods are now experiencing an increase is diabetes, heart disease, obesity, cancer, and degenerative disorders in addition to their original malnutrition? One study indicates the global rise in diabetes requires so much additional insulin that will be in short-supply by 2030 (Lapidus, 2018). And even animals are now experiencing human diseases.

Like pharmaceuticals, Americans need a Food Reference Manual that contains much the same information the Physician's Drug Reference manual (PDR), and Americans need more formal education about personal health, so the information in this book becomes common knowledge.

As a nurse and follower of Florence Nightingale's spirit, I believe we have identified the problems with health; now, it's time to intervene and reverse the symptoms. This book is intended to educate people about how food gets from our mouth into every cell in our body and how the quality of what we eat affects our overall health throughout our lifetime. Chapters may be read in any order. I hope readers also lookup my references for more details. My goal is to help everyone make better lifestyle choices, particularly with the foods we consume.

Over the past twenty-five years, food in America has dramatically changed. Many changes have increased the risks of illnesses for various individuals. Not all additives and GMO-foods harm everyone but knowing which ones are undermining your health and ability to feel the best you be is a good start.

The last chapter lists a few food additives and their potential side effects. These are just a few of the thousands of additives in our food. I hope this book inspires everyone to start investigating the additives in the foods frequently consumed and compare your health to the risks of those foods. If you experience any of the potential side effects, try eliminating those foods or additives for a few months to see if your symptoms disappear.

Be more aware of the food you buy, because food is intended to keep us healthy and not make us sick.

"God grant me the serenity to accept the things I cannot change; courage to change the things I can; and wisdom to know the difference," - Serenity Prayer

References

American Farm Bureau Federation. (2019). *Fast facts about agriculture.* Retrieved from American Farm Bureau Federation: https://www.fb.org/newsroom/fast-facts

Baron, C. (2019). *U.S. national health expenditure as a percent of GDP from 1960 to 2019.* Retrieved from Statista.com: https://www.statista.com/statistics/184968/us-health-expenditure-as-percent-of-gdp-since-1960/

Bethell, C. K. (2011). A national and state profile of leading health problems and health care quality for US children: key insurance disparities and across-state variations. *Academy of Pediatric Medicine*, S22-33.

Branum, A. L. (2008). *Food allergy among U.S. children: Trends in prevalence and hospitalizations.* Bethesda, MD: U.S. Dept. of health and human services; Center for Disease Control (CDC).

Buttorff, C, R. T. (2017). *Multiple chronic conditions in the United States.* Santa Monica, Ca: RAND.

CDC. (2007). *Overweight and Obesity Data: Childhood Overweight: Overweight Prevalence.* Retrieved from Centers for Disease Control and Prevention: http://www.cdc.gov/nccdphp/dnpa/obesity/childhood/prevalence.htm

CDC. (2017). *Health and economic costs of chronic diseases.* Retrieved from Center for Disease Control: https://www.cdc.gov/chronicdisease/about/costs/index.htm#ref1

Center for Medicare & Medicaid Services. (2017). *National health expenditure 2017 highlight.* Retrieved from Center for Medicare & Medicaid Services: https://www.cms.gov/Research-Statistics-Data-and-Systems/Statistics-Trends-and-Reports/NationalHealthExpendData/Downloads/highlights.pdf

Dabrowska, A. (2014). *Childhood Overweight and Obesity: Data Brief.* Congressional Research Service: R41420.

Daniels, K. (2012). *The soy-ling of America: second-hand soy from animal feeds.* Retrieved from The Western A. Foundation: https://www.westonaprice.org/health-topics/soy-alert/the-soy-ling-of-america-second-hand-soy-from-animal-feeds/

Hauck, D. (2014). *Supreme Court hands Monsanto victory over farmers on GMO seed patents, ability to sue.* Retrieved from USA News; Reuters: https://www.rt.com/usa/monsanto-patents-sue-farmers-547/

Jennifer. (2013). *Deaths caused by hidden soy in those with peanut allergies.* Retrieved from Healing Defined: http://healingredefined.org/peanut-soy-allergy-connection/

Lapidus, F. (2018). *Studies estimate a shortage of insulin by 2030.* Retrieved from Science & Health Broadcast: https://www.voanews.com/a/study-estimates-shortage-of-insulin-by-2030/4671590.html

NEL. (2012). *The food environment, eating out and body weight: A review of the evidence.* Retrieved from USDA; Nutrition evidence-based library, Nutrition insight 4: https://www.cnpp.usda.gov/sites/default/files/nutrition_insights_uploads/Insight 49. pdf

OECD. (2018). *Health spending.* Retrieved from Organization for Economic: https://data.oecd.org/

Onusic, S. (2013). *Violent Behavior: A solution in plain sight.* Retrieved from The Weston A. Price Foundation: https://www.westonaprice.org/health-topics/environmental-toxins/violent-behavior-a-solution-in-plain-sight/

Ormandy, E. D. (2011). Genetic engineering of animals: Ethical issues, including welfare concerns. *Canadian Veterinarian Journal, 52(5),* 544 - 550.

Porterfield, A. (2017). *Are GMOs responsible for a spike in food allergies?* Retrieved from Genetic Literacy Project: https://geneticliteracyproject.org/2017/09/13/gmos-responsible-spike-food-allergies/

Price, A. (2008). *Nutrition and Physical Degeneration; *8th Edition.* Le Mesa, Ca: Price-Pottenger Nutrition Foundation.

Rainer. (2018). *Why the Impossible Burger cannot be stopped.* Retrieved from Meat Alternatives: http://www.grubstreet.com/2018/04/impossible-foods-gets-more-funding-and-washington-lobbyist.html

Rose, M. (n.d.). *http://lawatlas.org/datasets/gmo-a1.* Retrieved from Temple University; Alawatlas.org: http://lawatlas.org/datasets/gmo-a1

Saitoh, S., Sato, T., Harada, H., & Takita, T. (2001). Transfer of soy isoflavone into the egg yolk of chickens. *Bioscience, Biotechnology, and Biochemistry, 65,* 2220-2225.

Scinta, W. (2016). *The history of portion sizes; how they have changed over the past decades.* Retrieved from Yourweightmatters.org.: https://www.yourweightmatters.org/portion-sizes-changed-time/

Spear, S. (2015). *DARK Act H. R. 1599.* Retrieved from EcoWatch: https://www.ecowatch.com/house-passes-dark-act-banning-states-from-requiring-gmo-labels-on-food-1882075093.html

Stevenson, H. . (2014). *Scientists use human genes in animals. So cows produce human-like milk - or do they.* Retrieved from GaiaHealth.com: http://gaia-health.com/environment/animals/scientists-use-human-genes-animals-cows-produce-human-like-milk/

Tonti-Filippini, N. (2001). *Ethics and human-animal transgenesis.* 1 - 13: L'Osservatore Romano supplement article.

WHO. (2018). Monitoring health for the SDGs, sustainable development goals, In T. W. Organization, *World Health Organization Assesses the World's Health Systems.* Geneva: The World Health Organization.

Yang B, W. J. (2011). *Characterization of Bioactive Recombinant Human Lysozyme Expressed in Milk of Cloned Transgenic Cattle.* Retrieved from PLoS ONE 6(3): e17593.: https://journals.plos.org/plosone/article?id=10.1371/journal.pone.0017593

Yang, H. Y. (2019). [Nutrition and food safety in China: problems, countermeasures, and prospects]. *53(3)*, 233-240.

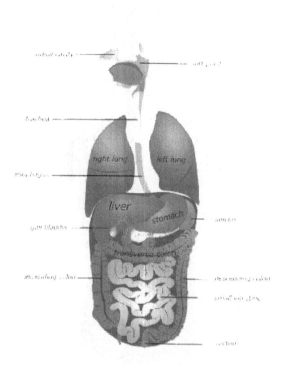

Chapter 1
The Digestive System

The digestive system, digestive tract, Gastro-Intestinal (GI) system, and Gastro-Intestinal tract are synonymous terms used interchangeably to describe the system that converts food into nutrients. Nutrients are then used to fuel all of our energy needs and build supplies, such as chemicals that are unique to each living thing.

The GI tract starts at the mouth and ends at the anus. In humans and other mammals, this system is made up of a series of structures that coordinate the processing of food, liquids, and pills through the GI tract. The walls of the entire GI system are coated with mucus to protect its lining from holes and deterioration. Multiple structures are comprised of muscles, whereas the stomach has the most. It's three layers of muscles are needed to churn everything into chyme. When a medication warns it may cause muscle weakness, few people think of their GI tract as a muscle, but food additives and medicines can affect our gastro-intestinal muscles in ways that impair our ability to swallow, digest and acquire nutrients necessary to sustain optimal health. A few examples of muscle weakness include difficulty swallowing, stomach muscles are too weak to churn food, and intestinal muscles fail to push food through our GI tract resulting in a blockage. The color and texture of our feces (stool) can tell us a lot about the efficiency of our digestive system.

Humans eat a wide range of plants and animals. Every time we put something into our mouth, we turn on our digestive system. The mechanical action of chewing, licking, and sucking use muscles in our mouth and throat. These actions stimulate physiological reactions to help break food into tiny particles that get sorted as macro and micronutrients. As those macro and micronutrients move down our assembly line of structures, food particles are filtered, categorized, and absorbed into the circulatory system, which uses our blood as a cargo system.

Every cell in our body needs specific nutrients. Inside cells are where nutrients get processed into supplies and ingredients and then packaged and delivered to organs throughout our body. The different organs need particular nutrients to make supplies necessary for those organs to function as intended and as a whole, make our bodies work well throughout our life.

Within the digestive system of all animals lives an entire microbiota eco-system. It is made up of trillions of microbes that aid in the digestion of food and keeping us healthy. They, too, act as an accessory organ but are an independent system that works like a sub-contractor.

Mechanical and physiological actions aided by our microbiota are equally important in the process of digestion. Mechanical structures + physiological actions + microbiota eco-system = digestion. When there is a problem with our digestive system, it can be either a physical malfunction in one of the mechanical structures or an imbalance in one or more of our physiological actions or something gone wrong with our microbiota.

Collectively they:

- ☺ Breakdown food and chemicals into tiny particles (nutrients)
- ☺ Push nutrients through the digestive system
- ☺ Sort, extract and package macro- & micronutrients to be sent where needed
- ☺ Cleanse nutrients before use: Filter toxins, neutralize harmful pollutants and poisons
- ☺ Provide energy to all cells and maintain enough in storage
- ☺ Provide ingredients to organs to build life-sustaining supplies
- ☺ Eliminate excess and unusable food particles

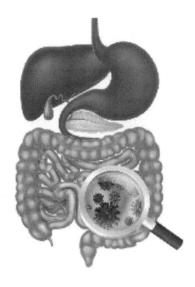

MECHANICAL STRUCTURES OF THE DIGESTIVE SYSTEM

Mechanical structures are the physical structures of our digestive system. Each act like hand-tools used to process food. These mechanical structures break food down into smaller particles starting with our teeth and tongue used to crush food into small particles, and then gravity pushes food, liquids, and other substances through our GI tract. Chewing also increases the surface area of the foods consumed. This makes the work of the rest of the GI tract easier. As the food gets pushed through the digestive system, it gets dismantled into a variety of macro- and micronutrients in preparation for use. Dismantled nutrients that are not needed immediately are either stored or eliminated.

The more thoroughly a person chews his or her food, the higher the number of nutrients are made available to be extracted. The more nutrients extracted, the quicker a person can feel satisfied from the food consumed. For this reason, many nutritionists recommend we chew every bite thoroughly, ten or more times, before swallowing. A healthy body will detect the amount of nutrients needed and send messages to and from the brain when enough has been consumed.

Many structures make up the digestive system. They are all connected, somewhat like an assembly line. As food is passing through our digestive system, a few accessory organs perform specific actions that are vital to the processing of nutrients. Accessory organs are kind of like sub-contractors. They are an independent organ that provides services to multiple systems. The liver, gallbladder, and pancreas are accessory organs that carry-out necessary actions in the digestive system.

Our kidneys are another organ in our body that aids in filtering toxins in addition to regulating chemical and fluid balance. Even though their functions affect the use of nutrients and are affected by what we consume, our kidneys are not physically connected to our digestive system, and therefore, they are not considered to be an accessory organ.

Structures of the Digestive System, Gastro-Intestinal (GI) tract:

The mouth:

- ☺ Chews and churns the food to crush into smaller particles
- ☺ Signals salivary glands to release enzymes for chemical Breakdown (a physiological action)
- ☺ Contains muscles in the cheeks, tongue, and gums
- ☺ Natural microbiota that resides on our mouth:
- ☺ Adhere to our teeth to prevent being swallowed
- ☺ Protect teeth from cavities; if harmful microbes enter gums and teeth, they can gain access to our blood and travel to other organs where they cause heart failure, cancer, Alzheimer's, diabetes, and other health problems, (Li, Systemic diseases caused by oral infections, 2000). Childhood oral infections and cavities are linked to adulthood heart disease and strokes. One study of 755 participants over 27 years has linked oral infections during childhood with carotid atherosclerosis in adulthood, (Pussinen, 2019).

Salivary glands:

- ☺ Moistens and lubricate food
- ☺ Breaks down food particles
- ☺ Arouses taste that stimulates appetite

Pharynx*:*

- ☺ Connects the mouth, nose, and esophagus
- ☺ Muscular accessory organ helps both the digestive and respiratory systems
- ☺ Causes the smell of good food to stimulate salivary glands or if bad, it can inhibit salivary gland secretion

Epiglottis:

- ☺ A mucous lined valve-like flap made of elastic cartilage
- ☺ Covers the trachea when food is swallowed, so to guide food into the stomach. It covers the esophagus when air is breathed in, which directs fresh oxygen into the lungs
- ☺ When we talk while eating, we swallow both air and food at the same time, which can confuse our epiglottis, causing the epiglottis to incorrectly close the tube to the stomach and open the tube to our lungs, thereby allowing food and liquid to pass into the lungs. This is how we choke on our food.
- ☺ Also, eating too fast can cause choking because the epiglottis may not have enough time between food and breathes to determine which tube to cover accurately.

Esophagus:

- ☺ A muscular tube that propels food to the stomach
- ☺ Lubricates food and its passageway

Stomach:

- ☺ The most muscular structure of the GI tract; made up of three kinds of muscles
  - o Contains stretch receptors in the layers of muscles that:
  - o Signals peristalsis to propel stomach contents into the intestines after food has been thoroughly broken down and mixed
  - o Signal the brain to stop eating when the stomach is too full
  - o Churns and combines food into smaller particles
- ☺ Mucous protects the stomach's lining and limits absorption
- ☺ Manufactures and secretes stomach acids: Hydrochloric Acids (HCI), potassium chloride (KCl) and sodium chloride (NaCl)

☺ Secretes intrinsic-factor needed to absorb vitamin B12 in the small intestine
☺ Activate stomach acids and enzymes (physiological actions) to:
   o Breakdown proteins into amino acids
   o Absorb fat-soluble substances
   o Disinfect and kill disease-causing microorganisms
   o Maintain pH balance at about 2.5

Liver:

☺ An accessory organ
☺ Before birth, it is the main site for embryonic hematopoiesis (development of bone marrow)
☺ Converts carbohydrates, fats, and proteins into organic particles that can be used to manufacture hormones, enzymes, Vitamin D and cholesterol
☺ Stores vitamins and iron
☺ Aids in producing new red blood cells
☺ Destroys old blood cells
☺ Filters chemicals and destroys poisons/toxins/ unhealthy microbes
☺ Filters out excessive proteins
☺ Processes medications and chemicals to be used in specific ways
☺ Assesses body's energy needs and produces cholesterol to meet those needs
☺ Contains receptor sites that attract Low-Density Cholesterol (LDL) out of the blood to restore or recycle worn-out lipids into bile to be stored in the gallbladder

Gallbladder:

☺ An accessory organ
☺ Produces bile salts that:
   o Emulsifies fat: Mix fat particles with bile salt to increase the use
   o Neutralizes stomach acid as chyme enters the small intestines
☺ Stores and concentrates bile
☺ Fats are not soluble in water. Before dietary fat can be digested, it must be emulsified. Bile emulsifies the fat we eat.
☺ The liver makes bile continuously and stores it in the gallbladder until it is needed. However, when too little fat is consumed, bile

remains in the gallbladder where it turns to sludge and forms into gallstones, (Festi D., 1998), (Groves, nd).

Pancreas:

☺ A glandular accessory organ that secretes its products into the GI tract
☺ Manufactures hormones that regulate:
  o Glucose
  o Fatty acid levels in the blood
  o Insulin
  o Glucagon
  o Appetite: Ghrelin, Leptin
☺ Manufacture enzymes that:
  o Neutralizes stomach acid
  o Process proteins into amino acids
  o Process carbohydrates, fats, and starches into energy

Small intestines:

☺ Made up of three consecutive mucous lined muscular tubes that connect the stomach to the large intestine:
  o Duodenum
  o Jejunum
  o Ileus
☺ 90% of digestion occurs in the small intestines; the other 10% occurs in the stomach and large intestines
☺ Completes processing of nutrients:
  o Neutralizes acidity from stomach contents (chyme)
  o Sends chyme to liver
  o Receives nutrients from liver, gallbladder, and pancreas
☺ Absorbs nutrients into the blood to be shipped to cells and organs
☺ Propels waste into the large intestines

Large intestines:

☺ Last part of the digestive system
☺ Like a garbage can, it collects waste such as worn-out blood cells and cholesterol particles, also unused processed meat and plants products

☺ Hosts majority of our microbiota that completes the Breakdown of food waste
☺ By absorbing water, it:
  o Concentrates the waste and temporarily stores it as feces
  o Excess fluid is sent to kidneys by way of our cargo system (blood)
  o Absorbs electrolytes, and vitamins produced by microbiota

Rectum:

☺ Stores and expels waste

Anus:

☺ The opening to eliminate unused byproducts (feces)

Kidneys are not a part of the digestive system, but they are responsible for:

☺ Filtering chemicals and toxins
☺ Filtering excessive protein
☺ Regulate the volume of fluid in our blood
☺ Regulate the acidity (pH balance) of our blood
☺ Eliminate excess fluid, chemicals, and toxins in our urine

Microbiota, Gut-Flora (See Chapter 2):

☺ An independent ecosystem living inside our GI system
☺ Helps digestion
☺ Prevent and reverses disease processes
☺ Unhealthy gut flora can weaken our digestive system and cause diseases
☺ Produce vitamin K, folate and Short-Chain Fatty Acids (SCFA)

PHYSIOLOGICAL MECHANISMS OF THE DIGESTIVE SYSTEM

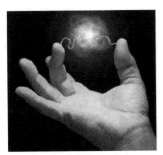

Internal Electricity

The physiological mechanisms provide electrical stimulation using electrolytes and chemical reactions to activate our enzymes and hormones. Our body produces its electrolytes, enzymes, and hormones from the food we eat. These compounds aid in the digestion of the food and are used to manufacture specific chemicals and supplies our body needs.

Electricity is needed to help food pass efficiently through the entire GI system using peristalsis. Electrolytes produce energy. Peristalsis is a series of wave-like contractions and relaxation of muscles that propel solids and liquids through the muscular tubes of the throat into the stomach and then throughout the intestines. All of our muscles use electrolytes for electrical stimulation, including those surrounding each organ in our body: Heart, lungs, stomach, and so forth. If your electrolytes are out of balance, it can turn off peristalsis in our digestive system.

When medical professionals use a stethoscope to listen to your stomach, they are listening for bowel sounds produced by peristalsis. Weak or no bowel sounds after eating a meal may indicate there may be a problem with our electrolytes, which is known as an ileus. Ileus occurs when there is no electricity sent to your stomach muscles. When this happens, food is unable to move throughout your GI tract. Without peristalsis, food can build-up, backup, and cause a blockage in the system.

Once food enters the mouth and chewing begins, the mechanical Breakdown of food activates enzyme-rich saliva, which is released in the mouth and begins the chemical activities. Chemical digestion uses enzymes to dismantle food particles. Saliva contains specialized enzymes known as salivary-amylase that breaks-down sugars, starches, carbohydrates, and fats into simple compounds that can be used later to build supplies.

When we swallow, peristalsis stimulates the muscles in our esophagus to contract and relax. This action propels food through the throat into the stomach. Our entire digestive system is made up of muscles.

Amylase is an enzyme manufactured and sent from the pancreas. Amylase only works in alkaline (non-acid) environments. Therefore, sugars and starches begin to Breakdown in the mouth but do not breakdown any further in the stomach. They wait until they reach the small intestines where additional amylase is secreted to complete its Breakdown.

The stomach is very acidic. This acid is needed for the enzyme pepsin to breakdown the proteins into amino acids and fats into fatty acids. Here is where fat-soluble substances such as alcohol and aspirin get absorbed (OpenStax CNX, 2018). Foods remain in the stomach until it becomes a thick soup-like mixture of decomposed nutrients known as chyme. More complex nutrients take longer to process, which can make a person feel full for more extended periods compare to processed foods that can be quickly decomposed and mixed into chyme.

As the processed contents of the stomach (known as chyme) is released into the small intestines, the gallbladder secrets bile into the small intestine to deactivate the stomach's acid. The pancreas also secretes amylase to complete the breakdown of sugar and starch.

The liver filters the chyme to remove toxins. It then extracts nutrients to be used by the liver to manufacture and recycle cholesterol while sorting the remaining chyme to be distributed to the pancreas, gallbladder, and small intestines. While the pancreas performed its activities, the small intestines absorb amino acids, lipids, nucleic acids, water, minerals, and vitamins into our blood (our cargo system) to be transported to other organs that manufacture more chemicals needed by the body.

Unused nutrients are pushed into the large intestine to complete the process and eliminate excess waste. Healthy microbiota in the large intestine performs chemical digestion that aids in immunity. Ions, water, minerals, vitamins, and organic particles get absorbed here. Once absorbed, these nutrients affect cell-reproduction and formation of every function of our body.

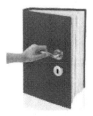

Key Points

♣ Mucus lines our digestive system to protects its lining and structure

♣ Most of the digestive system is made up of muscles. Weakened muscles can result in difficulty swallowing, digesting foods and eliminating unused food particles

♣ Our liver and kidneys filter food, chemicals, and toxins

♣ When there is too little fat in the diet, the unused bile builds up and sits in the gall bladder; Bile buildup can eventually turn into gallstones

♣ Mechanical structures break-down nutrients to be absorbed into the body's cells and blood

♣ Inside our blood are cells that process and package nutrients

♣ Nutrients are like ingredients that each organ in the body uses to make supplies

♣ Our digestive system uses three primary mechanisms: Mechanical structures + physiological system + our microbiota = our digestive system

♣ The physiological actions provide electricity to our mechanical structures

♣ Electric impulses help make the muscles in our digestive system work

♣ Peristalsis is a series of wave-like contractions and relaxation of muscles that propel solids and liquids through the muscular tubes of the throat and throughout the intestines

♣ Foods and medications that warn of potential muscle weakness may cause difficulty with swallowing and digesting food because our digestive system is made up of many muscles

♣ Our physiological mechanisms include hormones, enzymes, and electrolytes, all of which make up the chemical reactions needed to breakdown, reassemble, and use of nutrients in our body

Rebekah S. Mead

References

Festi, D., C. A. (1998). Gallbladder motility and gallstone formation in obese patients following very-low-calorie diets. Use it (fat) to lose it (well). *International Journal of Obesity Metabolic Disorders, 22(6)*, 592-600.

Groves, B. (nd). *Dietary Causes of* Gallstones *Information.* Retrieved from Second.opinions.co.uk: http://www.second-opinions.co.uk/gallstones.html#.XEcacvZFyH8

Li, X. K. (2000). Systemic diseases caused by oral infections. *Clinical Microbiology Review, 13(4)*, 547-558.

OpenStax CNX. (2018). *Chemical Digestions and Absorption: A closer look.* Retrieved from Anatomy and Physiology: Module 7 Digestive system: https://courses.lumenlearning.com/suny-ap2/chapter/chemical-digestion-and-absorption-a-closer-look/

Pussinen, P. P.-K. (2019). Association of childhood oral infections with cardiovascular risk factors and subclinical atherosclerosis in adulthood. *JAMA Network.*

Chapter 2

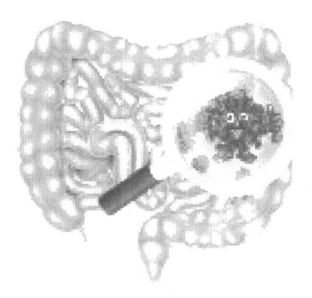

Our Unique Microbiota (Gut Flora)

Our microbiota is a complex interdependent ecosystem that co-exists within the digestive system of all animals. It is an independent ecosystem made up of trillions of bacteria, fungus, protozoa, and viruses that share the food and chemicals we consume (Jockers, 2014). Like an accessory organ or sub-contractor, it provides benefits that are essential to our life, whereas each organism has its own genes that control its own destiny.

This independent eco-system plays a crucial role in our overall wellbeing (homeostasis). Inside our GI tract, they "act like a huge chemical factory that helps to digest food, regulate hormones, excrete toxins, produce healing compounds and keep your gut healthy," (Chalkboard, 2018). Our microbiota protects against infections and diseases by directly fighting off invading microbes and by orchestrating appropriate immune responses, (Becattini, 2016).

This ecosystem thrives on our environmental exposures and the foods we eat. Everything we breathe, absorb, inject, or ingest affects the makeup of our microbiota. All animals, including humans, are born with a sterile gut that quickly evolves in response to its environment. Microbiota is created and rebuilt throughout life. Therefore, it is strongly affected by our cultural values and where we live. In other words, the microbes in our digestive system evolve from exposure to the foods we choose to eat and where we live, all of which are lifestyle choices. Because of the wide variety of lifestyle choices available on this planet, the makeup of everyone's microbiota is thought to be as unique to each person as fingerprints (GMNW, 2015).

Our gut-flora communicates with our brain and other organs. "Emerging evidence suggests there is a bidirectional interaction between the intestinal microbiota and the brain. This crosstalk may play a substantial role in neurologic diseases, including anxiety, depression, autism, multiple sclerosis, Parkinson's disease, and Alzheimer's disease" (Cox L. W., 2018). When our gut microorganisms detect a change in its environment that threatens the existence of its social network, it communicates with our organs to help accommodate its needs. The messages sent by our microbiota either stimulate or inhibit the production of hormones, enzymes, immune cells, and other supplies. They influence just about every function, including weight, cholesterol, and fertility. The quality of our microbiota ecosystem strongly influences the development and function of our central nervous system, management of insulin, and even our personality. In fact, our gut flora is so essential to our immune system for the prevention and reversal diseases that some scientists claim that gut-flora has become a "forgotten organ" (Quigley, 2013), (Cheema, 2016), (Wu, 2012). Many medical professionals overlook the health-status of gut-flora when ruling-out the root cause of symptoms, whereas correcting the health of the gut may prevent or reverse a disease process.

"The intestinal microbiota has become a relevant aspect of human health. Microbial colonization runs in parallel with immune system maturation and plays a role in intestinal physiology and regulation. Increasing evidence on early microbial contact suggests that human intestinal microbiota is seeded before birth. Maternal microbiota forms the first microbial environment, and from birth, the microbial diversity increases and converges toward an adult-like microbiota by the end of the first 3–5 years of life. Perinatal factors such as mode of delivery, diet, genetics, and intestinal mucin glycosylation all contribute to influencing microbial colonization. Once established, the composition of the gut microbiota is relatively stable throughout adult life but can change as a result of bacterial infections, antibiotic treatment, lifestyle, surgical, and a long-term change in diet. Shifts in this complex microbial system have been reported to increase the risk of disease. Therefore, an adequate establishment of microbiota and its maintenance throughout life would reduce the risk of disease in early and late-life. This review discusses recent studies on the early colonization and factors influencing this process, which impact health" (Rodríguez, 2015).

"Humans have co-evolved with the intestinal microbiota, and this long-term relationship is maintained by regulatory factors that help select for a beneficial microbiota. The bidirectional immune, endocrine, and neural signaling pathways establish a mechanism for homeostatic communication between the microbiota and the CNS. The interaction between the brain and the intestinal microbiota plays an important role in mood, metabolism, cognition, and motor function. Disruptions in the microbiota-gut-brain axis can contribute to a variety of diseases, including anxiety, depression, MS, PD, and autism. A better understanding of which microbial components, directly and indirectly, signal to the brain could provide promising new targets for treating neurologic diseases" (Weerth, 2017).

In nature, when plants or animals die, some microorganisms thrive on the dead tissues. These microorganisms are nature's way of cleaning up the earth. But, when those microbes enter a healthy body, they can cause a lot of harm by starting the process of destruction and death. Healthy gut flora will attempt to get rid of them by an army of immune cells designed to kill each kind of bad-microbe that enters our body. If harmful microbes do take over and win-the-battle, they need a new environment to reproduce and survive, which requires changes to our digestive system.

This new environment is usually inconsistent with our health. The way they impose their lifestyle may include sending revised messages to our brain and other organs. Their further instructions may involve a design that creates diseases that lead to premature death. When harmful microbes start to impose their lifestyle on our body, we may initially feel vague symptoms such as nausea, weakness, or a host of other mild symptoms. A change in the color, odor, and texture of our feces may be early signs that something inside our gut is changing for the worse. If not stopped, those harmful microbes begin to replace health gut microbes and then multiply until they over-throw and impair the entire digestive system or other organs and structures.

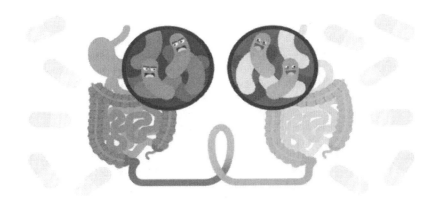

While the use of antibiotics has benefits, their over-use harms our healthy gut flora. "Antibiotics alter the microbiota composition, resulting in an increased risk of disease, secondary infections, allergy, and obesity. Antibiotics also help the spread of drug-resistant pathogens (Becattini, 2016).

There are many ways for harmful microbes to gain access to our digestive system:

☺ Malnutrition nutrition / Poor or Unhealthy diet

☺ Pollution in the Environment: Air, water, land, mental stress, etc.

☺ Insufficient sunlight

☺ Smoking cigarettes, marijuana, and other chemicals

☺ Medications that have adverse side-effects

☺ Trans-genetic replication

Dietary habits, exercise, sleep, and environmental exposures play significant roles in influencing the quality of gut microbiota. Too much or too little of each nutrient will impact the ability of our microbiota to carry out its functions. When our microbiota is at its best, our immune system not only prevents disease but by detoxifying our gut, it can repair and restore our body (Jockers, 2014).

Unhealthy gut-flora often causes inflammation along the GI tract, which is known to progress into a variety of autoimmune diseases such as Rheumatoid Arthritis, diabetes, asthma allergies and celiac disease, (Wu, 2012). The development of unhealthy microbiota during early childhood may be a critical determinant of disease expression in later life (Quigley, 2013).

Tooth decay can enter the blood system, carrying harmful microbes to other organs where it can cause various childhood diseases or fester for decades resulting in chronic diseases or weakened organs and bones.

An overgrowth of unhealthy gut-flora leads often leads to Inflammatory Bowel Diseases (IBD) and Irritable Bowel Syndrome (IBS), which have been identified as the initial cause of many chronic health conditions such as heart disease, metabolic syndrome, Alcoholic Liver Disease (ALD), Non-Alcoholic Fatty Liver Disease (NAFLD), cirrhosis and cancer, (Quigley, 2013) (Swidinski, 2005), (Baohong, 2017).

Our gut microbiota has widespread influence over ingested pharmaceutical products (medications). Challenges of actually getting the intended benefits of any medication depend on the health of our digestive system and our microbiota. Previous research shows the powerful influence microbiota has on how and where those medications get absorbed, all of which affect its actions on our body. Therefore, the effectiveness of your prescribed drugs is strongly influenced by the health of your microbiota, "which is too often under-appreciated by medical professionals treating various conditions" (Enright, 2016). Treating an unhealthy microbiota and digestive system before or in addition to taking medications may be in your best interest. There are many known medications to which the health of our microbiota and digestive system influences its effectiveness: (Enright, 2016):

- ☺ Antineoplastic Medicines
- ☺ Cardiovascular Medicines
- ☺ Central Nervous System Active Medicine
- ☺ Immunosuppressant Medicines
- ☺ Antacids
- ☺ Antidepressants

Antibiotic treatments, vaccinations, and sterile hygiene practices can also harm your gut microbiota composition (Wu, 2012). When exposed to something harmful, your healthy microbiota can attack and consume harmful microbes. They send signals to your organs to increase the production of supplies needed to fight off illnesses. Taking medication such as antibiotics may inadvertently kill off your healthy gut bacteria because most of your microbiota is made up of many different kinds of bacteria in which antibiotics do not pick and choose which bacteria to destroy. By killing off the healthy bacteria, this may consequently hinder your ability to build immunity and fight off chronic conditions while making way for harmful microbes to take over.

The growth of unhealthy and unnatural gut floral may then be the underlying cause of someone's inability to prevent and repair their body. Children in America today are exposed to many food additives and chemicals that did not exist in our food thirty years ago. Many additives and pesticides used in our food today contain DNA that disrupts the natural activity of plant and animal hormones. When children consume these foods, their evolving microbiota is exposed to the food additives and pesticides that are intended to destroy Mother Nature, which all of us are a part of. For instance, many pesticides are hormone disruptors that are used to prevent seed fertility and therefore prevent farmers from saving the seeds for use in another season. When humans consume the produce sprayed with those hormone disruptors, their hormones can also be disrupted by those pesticides.

Older adults are similarly at risk. The development of our microbiota is an ongoing process that continually evolves with each exposure in life. So even if someone has eaten a particular food or taken a specific medication for many years, our gut-flora can be changed by a new environmental exposure in such a way as to change how we react to those foods and drugs in the future.

Researchers for a long time have recognized the many potentially opposing interactions between human microbiota and medications, including the development of a new disease while a patient is treated for other problems. An unhealthy microbiome can result in adverse drug reactions. Researchers, long before 2009, foresaw treatment of gut bacteria as playing a crucial role in the prevention and treatment of most mental and physical ailments, (Clayton, 2009).

Since1996, scientifically manipulated seeds and transgenetic animals created in laboratories have replaced much of our organic-based agriculture and farm-raised animals (FDA, 2008). Many foods sold in the supermarkets today contain Genetically Modified Organisms (GMO) and trans-genetic or cloned animals.

One example of an unintended consequence of gene manipulation is peanut butter, which has easily cross-contaminated by GMO soy. Before the introduction of GMO crops, peanut butter and jelly sandwiches were a healthy lunch for many children over many generations. Nutrient-rich organic peanuts have no cholesterol (because they come from a plant) and are high in fiber. Organic-natural peanuts are high in protein. It also has healthy fat that gives us energy and helps build our hormones and immune system, and it is high in vitamin B6 and the mineral magnesium. Then came the new GMO oils. Highly allergenic but a cheap additive. Many modern peanut butter producers now replace the natural oils in peanut butter with other less expensive oils.

Between 1997 until 2002, just five years, peanut allergies in American children doubled (Sicherer SH, 2003).

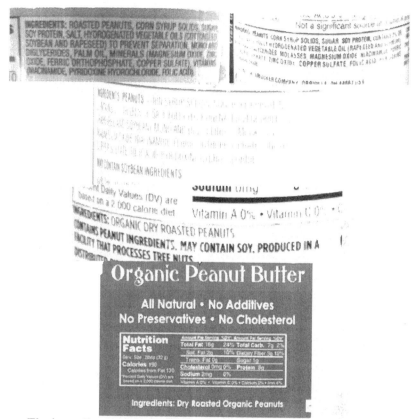

The ingredients vary significantly in the wide variety of brands of peanut butter sold in the USA

Compared to countries where the cultivation and sale of GMO products are banned, the incidence of food allergies, including peanuts, is much higher in the USA. For instance, in Asia and Africa, which are only two of many such countries that ban many GMO crops (Sustainable Pulse, 2015) (Genetic Literacy Project, 2010), peanuts are still a staple food and a vital source for healthy protein. "It is interesting that their peanut allergies, as well as other food allergies, are much less than in the USA. In fact, peanut-based foods have a 90% success rate in treating newborns and infants for health and growth purposes" (PeanutInstitute.org, Unk).

It does appear that the GMO oils and other ingredients added to peanut butter has had unintended consequence causing many young children today to be allergic to peanuts and peanut butter. Ultimately, GMO crops have denied American children one enjoyable source of protein. As for those who attribute their allergy solely to peanuts, they may be experiencing allergic reactions to other foods containing the same GMO oils. Consumers and parents may be falsely blaming peanut dust or food handlers for their allergic-reactions when soy oils may very well be the real culprit. Soy-based oils are added to everything from hamburgers to salad dressings (Segedie, 2019).

The good news is that our microbiota is continuously evolving to adjust to its environment. What this means is, if a food additive, chemical, or environmental exposure is making you sick, your body can repair itself by eliminating those harmful exposures and feeding your gut healthy foods to help regrow your healthy microbiota in our gut.

Some medical providers have even resorted to fecal transplants to restore healthy gut flora.

FYI
If your organic peanut butter is too hard to spread, try blending a chunk with a small amount of healthy coconut or avocado oil. It will then spread easy

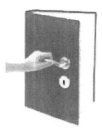

Key Points

♣ There are trillions of microorganisms living inside our bodies. Their ecosystem lives throughout our entire digestive system.

♣ Microorganisms in our digestive system help digest food, produce vitamins, regulate hormones, excrete toxins, and produce healing compounds that keep your gut healthy.

♣ Diets that occlude certain nutrients or lack a variety of nutrients can cause malnutrition. Over long periods, these diets can cause deficiencies and harmful changes in the body's microbiota.

♣ Harmful microorganisms can invade our GI system and impair our gut flora.

♣ Healthy microbiota can prevent and even reverse diseases.

♣ Allergies to Genetically Modified Soy oils are common. GMO soy easily cross-contaminates with other GMO plants, especially peanuts. Therefore, anyone allergic to GMO soy will experience the same allergic reaction to those other plants. Many peanut butter brands add soy oil and other soy derivatives. An allergic reaction to GMO soy may mistakenly be attributed to the peanut butter.

♣ The health status of a persons' microbiota can have a strong influence on the effectiveness of prescribed medications.

♣ Antibiotics can kill off the healthy bacteria in a gut, making it easier for harmful bacteria to take over.

♣ Tooth decay can cause heart valve failure.

♣ A change in my lifestyle, such as moving to a new location, can cause a person to react differently to foods and medications they have consumed for many years.

References

Becattini, S. T. (2016). Antibiotic-Induced changes in the Intestinal microbiota and disease. *Trends of Molecular Medicine, 22 (6)*, 458 - 478.

Chalkboard. (2018). *7 Changes that will improve your gut.* Retrieved from Chalkboard: https://thechalkboardmag.com/7-diet-changes-to-improve-gut-health-for-life

Cheema, A. K. (2016). Chemopreventative metabolites are related with change in intestinal measured at A-T mice and decreased carcinogenesis. *PLoS*, 1 - 19.

Clayton, T. B. (2009). Pharmacometabonomic identification of a significant host-microbiome metabolic interaction affecting human drug metabolism. *Proceedings of the National Academy of Sciences of the USA, 106 (34)*, 14728-14733.

Cox, L. W. (2018). Microbiota signaling pathways that influence neurologic disease. *Journal of Neurotherapeutics, 15(1)*, 135-145.

Enright, E. G. (2016). The Impact of the gut microbiota on drug metabolism and clinical outcome. *Yale Journal of Biologic Medicine, v89*, 375-382.

FDA. (2008). *Animal cloning: A risk assessment.* Rockville, MD: Center for Veterinary Medicine, Food and Drug Administration; Dept of Human Services.

Genetic Literacy Project. (2010). *Where are GMO crops and animals approved and banned?* Retrieved from Genetic Literacy Project: https://gmo.geneticliteracyproject.org/FAQ/where-are-gmos-grown-and-banned/

GMNW. (2015). *Your microbiota is as unique as your fingerprints.* Retrieved from Gut Microbiota News Watch (GMNW): https://www.gutmicrobiotaforhealth.com/en/your-microbiome-is-like-a-unique-fingerprint/

PeanutInstitute.org. (Unk). *Peanut allergy: White paper.* Retrieved from PeanutInstitute.org.: http://www.peanut-institute.org/resources/downloads/peanut_allergy_whitepaper.pdf

Quigley, E. (2013). Gut bacteria in health and disease. *Gastroenterology and Hepatology, 9(9)*, 560 -569.

Rodriguez, J. M. (2015). The composition of the gut microbiota throughout life, with an emphasis on early life. *Journal of Microb Ecol Health Disease, 26*, Published online 2015 Feb 2. DOI: 10.3402/mehd.v26.26050.

Segedie, L. (2019). *There's WHAT in My Sandwich? Detoxing Unhealthy Peanut Butter.* Retrieved from Mamavation: https://www.mamavation.com/featured/detoxing-unhealthy-peanut-butters.html

Sicherer SH, M.-F. A. (2003). Prevalence of peanut and tree nut allergy in the United States determined by means of a random digit dial telephone survey: a 5-year follow-up study. *Journal of Clinical Immunology, 112(6)*, 1203-1207.

Sustainable Pulse. (2015). *GMO crops now banned in 39 countries.* Retrieved from Sustainable Pulse: https://sustainablepulse.com/2015/10/22/gm-crops-now-banned-in-36-countries-worldwide-sustainable-pulse-research/#.XJfS9XdFyH8

Weerth, C. (2017). Do bacteria shape our development? Crosstalk between intestinal microbiota and HPA axis. *Journal of Neuroscience & Biobehavioral Reviews,v.83*, 458-471.

Wu, H. W. (2012). The role of gut microbiota in immune homeostasis and autoimmunity. *Gut Microbes V3(1)*, 4-14.

Chapter 3

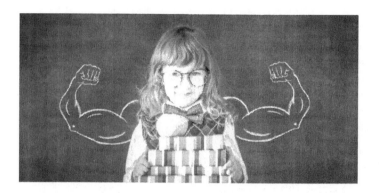

The Fate of Food: From Our Mouth into Our Cells

The goal of digestion is to get nutrients from our mouths into our cells. What we consume generates energy and manufacture supplies in quantities sufficient enough to support all mental and physical functions of the body. Even as we sleep, our body is continually using power to manufacture chemicals and putting them into action.

Everything that enters our mouth gets broken down into many tiny nutrient particles. The process of eating is like taking a car apart right down to its last bolt. What we ingest becomes the building blocks and ingredients used to make all of the energy and chemicals our body needs. Our digestive system sorts filters and assembles these building blocks into energy and chemicals our body uses in various ways. Some nutrient-particles are used by the digestive system, while others get packaged up and loaded into our blood to get circulated (transported) to other organs. Upon delivery, those nutrient-particles get assembled into different supplies unique to those organs.

Nutrients get absorbed into cells where they are processed. Whereas, our blood acts like a cargo system that delivers oxygen and nutrients to every organ and brings back the worn-out blood cells, cholesterol, and other particles. Humans have millions of cells. Each cell is made up of trillions of more molecules. These molecules are what regulate every function of our body so to sustain our life.

The quality of our diet dramatically influences our ability to build and maintain a healthy brain and body from the cradle to the grave. Every morsel of food, food additive, and chemical put into our mouth become building blocks that can generate, enhance, or inhibit our mechanical, microbiota, and physiological functions. The food and chemicals we consume either make or break our ability to prevent diseases and injuries. What we ingest can build a community of healthy microbiota or grow cancerous tumors; it can keep us fertile or make us infertile; it can keep us vital with energy or deplete our ability to enjoy life. Therefore, the quality of nutrients put into our body dramatically influences our health and is more important than quantity.

Not all nutrients are created equal; the lower the quality and variety, the poorer one's health will be or become. Obesity in America has become the leading cause of diabetes and heart disease. Obesity is due to more calories consumed than the body can burn off, while diabetes and heart disease are due to malnutrition (Via, 2012), (García, 2009). According to one endocrinologist, "Despite excessive dietary consumption, obese individuals have high rates of micronutrient deficiencies" (Via, 2012). Simply put, consuming large quantities of foods that are full of empty calories causes malnutrition and obesity.

When nutrient-rich food breaks down into tiny particles, its nutrients become "bioavailable." Some of those bioavailable nutrients get processed and absorbed. Organic foods high bioavailability can be relied upon to get the right amount of nutrients our body needs. Those that have poor bioavailability produce lesser quality energy, hormone, enzyme, neurotransmitter, or other supplies, and may get stored as fat. If you're lucky, your body will eliminate them.

Many excess calories from the proteins, carbohydrates, and fats consumed are converted to fat and stored. Stored fat is how our body reserves energy and nutrients for future use. Quality is a crucial factor. When people eat foods that contain harmful additives and chemical residues over many years, those chemicals can build up in their body fat. As those people lose weight or breastfeed, their bodies use the stored fat. Any stored chemicals are then brought back into their blood and possibly in more concentrated forms (WDHS, 2018).

Whether specific foods have high, mediocre, or poor bioavailability depends on multiple factors:

☺ Types of food: Some foods are nutrient-dense, meaning most of the calories contain one or more nutrients. Those that are nutrient-deprived have calories with no or very little nutrient value.

☺ Organic foods consistently have specific nutrients. All organic apples contain the same basic nutrients; All organic cows produce cow's milk that has similar nutrients.

Products of Biotechnology (POB) may:

☹ Add or remove genes to create unique traits

☹ Have chemical residues or genes that resist or destroy microorganisms

☹ Resemble a beef hamburger but be genetically modified soybeans with genes to make it look and bleed like a real burger. The nutrient values are not the same. Soy burgers are higher in calories, sodium, and saturated fat with less protein (Yu, 2018). Those who are allergic to genetically altered or organic soy would greatly benefit from the full disclosure of ingredients, including what DNA mutation was added to that particular soy.

☹ Depending on the amount consumed, some food additives and chemicals, including medications, can:
  o Prevent or increase absorption and usage of nutrients
  o Change the way your body reacts to nutrients, e.g.. You feel hungry after eating a meal instead of feeling full
  o When a nutrient is highly "bioavailable," we can depend on them to be digested and absorbed with a high percentage of success. "When a nutrient is said to have poor bioavailable, its digestion, absorption, or both can be much more difficult to absorb and much less predictable" (Mateljan, 2019).

By choosing organic foods that are dependably high in bioavailability, we use our calories wisely, which will keep our bodies fit. Dependably nutrient-rich food is especially important during times of illness or healing from injuries. Choosing foods known for its high bioavailability is especially essential during childhood while their bodies are developing. The same is true for older adults who are more prone to memory problems and weakness.

What, when, and how we eat makes a difference. Specific nutrients consumed at various points in the day affect cognition, energy levels, and even social behavior. Multiple studies show a breakfast high in carbs without protein can lower one's ability to feel compassion for others, whereas a breakfast high in protein leads to friendlier attitudes throughout the day (Strang, 2017).

All animals convert food into nutrients used to support their body's needs regardless of whether it is human, domestic or wildlife, or fish. What each animal consumes affects the quality of their body. The quality of meat, dairy products, and eggs produced for human consumption is greatly affected by the quality of nutrients those animals consume. For example, mass-produced genetically-altered featherless chickens housed in over-crowded factory cages neither graze on a variety of organic plants or scratch for bugs. Instead, they consume a scientific diet of grain-pellets that may very likely come from cow manure (Owens, 1999). They lack exercise, sunlight, and the variety of healthy nutrients needed to build healthy, viable hormones, amongst other life-sustaining nutrients. The quality of their eggs and meat are the result of their poor lifestyle. Due to their crowded living conditions, many factory-grown chickens often receive antibiotics and other medications to prevent the spread of diseases caused by an over-crowded pen (Peachman, 2018), (USDA, 2015), which is passed on to the consumer.

Is it any wonder why Americans are confused when media reports news warning that eggs can increase unhealthy cholesterol levels and then at a later date announce that eggs are an excellent source of healthy cholesterol and much-needed protein?

Well, both reports are accurate because neither explains why. Chickens digest the foods they consume. Those foods breakdown into the nutrients used to build their enzymes, hormones, and other manufactured supplies needed to sustain their life.

Chickens that roam freely in a barnyard and fed only organic grains lead relatively stress-free lives. They get plenty of fresh air and sunlight. As a result, the hormones their bodies manufacture from the food they eat will produce eggs rich in healthy cholesterol and protein. Whereas, factory-raised featherless chickens living in crowded conditions and fed manure and medication, will manufacture hormones that produce eggs with low-quality nutrients.

One of my life's lessons was greatly affected by chicken eggs. I grew up on a farm with chickens and then raised my own after I got married. I loved to bake delicious, nutritious meals, and treats using fresh eggs from those hens.

Each Christmas, I baked a Black Forest cake using egg-whites whipped into a thick aerated creamy meringue. Other months I freshly baked lemon meringue pies with tall, fluffy peaks of meringue.

Shortly after I stopped farming and sold all my chickens, I relied on store-bought ingredients. Unbeknownst to me, the quality of eggs purchased in the store was changing. Around 2004, I was frequently disappointed when I couldn't beat egg whites into fluffy mounds of meringue. Also, eggs ran like water in a frying pan. I couldn't even get an omelet to stick together; they all turned out as burnt pieces of mush. All of my cherished old recipes were turning out flat and tasteless. Not only that, they were making me painfully bloated and fat. Sometimes my gallbladder throbbed for hours after a meal. Other times my tongue swelled up and hurt from a little-known condition called geographic tongue. Foods were changing in America without our knowledge. What I didn't know was making me sick, both mentally and physically.

I finally realized farm-raised chicken eggs not only looked and tasted different than those from featherless, frugally-fed caged chickens, they also produced very different nutrients. By switching to only eggs from organic-fed cage-free chickens, my favorite old recipes were once again rich in texture, flavor, and nutrients. The change was miraculous.

Through evidence-based research and experience, I began to realize not all food and additives are created equal. Allergies and food sensitivities to specific foods, additives, and pesticide residues may be responsible for physical and emotional reactions that are not typically associated with food. Confusion, mental blocking, dullness, lethargy, tenseness, irritability, dissociation, and perceptual distortions are some of the more common central nervous system allergic responses that individuals and their medical providers may not consider as food-related. The more I used real organic ingredients, the better my recipes turned out, and ultimately, my anxiety levels dropped. I feel more satisfied with less food, and neither my tongue nor stomach aches after meals the way they do when I eat processed food from unknown sources.

Getting back to the difference that quality makes, when food enters the mouth, it stimulates the chewing reflex, which activates the release of chemicals. The hormone insulin is secreted to make sure there is enough energy (sugar) in the blood to perform all the body's functions. Our insulin is also responsible for removing the excess units of energy from the blood by sending it to the pancreas to be stored as fat.

Our tongue and cheeks release enzymes during the initial phase of eating, which begins the process of breaking down food into as many tiny nutrient-molecules as possible. The more we chew, the greater exposure there is to the surface area of the nutrient-molecules, making more nutrients available. Therefore, thoroughly chewing every bite of food, ten or more times before swallowing, helps produce more nutrients that your body will use to build its supplies. By chewing thoroughly, more nutrients are available from less food. When our brain detects enough nutrients sufficient to meet the needs of our body, it will tell us to stop eating.

Natural foods contain multiple nutrients. By eating a variety of fresh fruits and vegetables in addition to high quality lean meats, milk and eggs, it is very possible to consume less food and still get all the necessary nutrients needed to manufacture the right quantity of enzymes, hormones, neurotransmitters, electrolytes, red blood cells and other internally produced supplies essential to sustain a long healthy life.

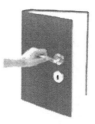

Key Points

♣ The goal of eating is to get nutrients and energy to every cell in our body.

♣ Everything we eat gets broken down into particles our body uses to make supplies. These particles become the ingredients and building-blocks used to make our enzymes, hormones, cholesterol, neurotransmitters, and other vital supplies.

♣ Every morsel of food, food additive, and chemical consumed (ingested) become building blocks that can generate, enhance, or inhibit our mechanical, microbiota, and physiological functions.

♣ All foods are *not* created equal; When the DNA of an apple is changed, its nutrient values and other qualities also change.

♣ Bioavailability measures how easily food releases its nutrients.

♣ Foods that have high bioavailability are nutrient-dense (it has many easy to use nutrients), which gives a body more nutrients per calorie.

♣ The more a person chews his or her food, the more nutrients that a person gets from each bite of food.

♣ By eating a variety of foods, our body can consume enough nutrition to stay healthy.

♣ No one grain or plant can provide all the nutrients needed by a body.

References

Becattini, S. T. (2016). Antibiotic-Induced changes in the Intestinal microbiota and disease. *Trends of Molecular Medicine, 22 (6)*, 458 - 478.

Chalkboard. (2018). *7 Changes that will improve your gut.* Retrieved from Chalkboard: https://thechalkboardmag.com/7-diet-changes-to-improve-gut-health-for-life

Cheema, A. K. (2016). Chemopreventative metabolites are related with change in intestinal measured at A-T mice and decreased carcinogenesis. *PLoS*, 1 - 19.

FDA. (2008). *Animal cloning: A risk assessment.* Rockville, MD: Center for Veterinary Medicine, Food and Drug Administration; Dept of Human Services.

Festi, D., C. A. (1998). Gallbladder motility and gallstone formation in obese patients following very-low-calorie diets. Use it (fat) to lose it (well). *International Journal of Obesity Metabolic Disorders, 22(6)*, 592-600.

García, O. L. (2009). Impact of micro deficiency on obesity. *Nutrition Review, 67 (10)*, 559 - 572.

Genetic Literacy Project. (2010). *Where are GMO crops and animals approved and banned?*Retrieved from Genetic Literacy Project: https://gmo.geneticliteracyproject.org/FAQ/where-are-gmos-grown-and-banned/

GMNW. (2015). *Your microbiota is as unique as your fingerprints.* Retrieved from Gut Microbiota News Watch (GMNW): https://www.gutmicrobiotaforhealth.com/en/your-microbiome-is-like-a-unique-fingerprint/

Groves, B. (nd). *Dietary Causes of Gallstones Information.* Retrieved from Second.opinions.co.uk: http://www.second-opinions.co.uk/gallstones.html#.XEcacvZFyH8

Mateljan, G. (2019). *What is bioavailability?* Retrieved from The George Mateljan Foundationwhfood.org: http://whfoods.org/genpage.php?tname=dailytip&dbid=305

PeanutInstitute.org. (Unk). *Peanut allergy: White paper.* Retrieved from PeanutInstitute.org.: http://www.peanut-institute.org/resources/downloads/peanut_allergy_whitepaper.pdf

Quigley, E. (2013). Gut bacteria in health and disease. *Gastroenterology and Hepatology, 9(9),* 560 -569.

Segedie, L. (2019). *There's WHAT in My Sandwich? Detoxing Unhealthy Peanut Butter.* Retrieved from Mamavation:
https://www.mamavation.com/featured/detoxing-unhealthy-peanut-butters.html

Sicherer SH, M.-F. A. (2003). Prevalence of peanut and tree nut allergy in the United States determined by means of a random digit dial telephone survey: a 5-year follow-up study. *Journal of Clinical Immunology, 112(6),* 1203-1207.

Strang, S. H. (2017). *Impact of nutrition on social decision making.* Retrieved from Proceedings of the National Academy of Sciences in the USA (PNAS):
https://www.pnas.org/content/114/25/6510

Sustainable Pulse. (2015). *GMO crops now banned in 39 countries.* Retrieved from SustainablePulse: https://sustainablepulse.com/2015/10/22/gm-crops-now-banned-in-36-countries-worldwide-sustainable-pulse-research/#.XJfS9XdFyH8

USDA. (2015). *The meat and poultry labeling terms.* Retrieved from the United States The Department of Agriculture:
https://www.fsis.usda.gov/wps/portal/fsis/topics/food-safety-education/get-answers/food-safety-fact-sheets/food-labeling/meat-and-poultry-labeling-terms/meat-and-poultry-labeling-terms/!ut/p/a1/jZFRb9owFIX_Cn3AL8zYSQiklawqSjdR1oZWsDXkpXIcJ7FI7NQ2o O7XL1B16

Via, M. (2012). The malnutrition of obesity: Micronutrient deficiencies that promote diabetes. *ISRN Endocrinology,* 103472.

Wu, H. W. (2012). The role of gut microbiota in immune homeostasis and autoimmunity. *Gut Microbes V3(1),* 4-14.

Yu, C. (2018). *Is the impossible burger really better for you than a regular burger?* Retrieved from Women's Health:
https://www.womenshealthmag.com/food/a21050196/the-impossible-burger/

Chapter 4

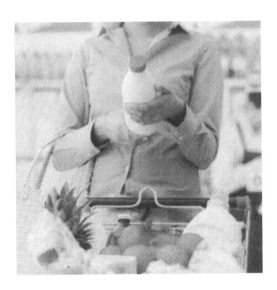

Quality In = Quality Out

"Let Food Be Thy Medicine," Hippocrates

Our body needs a variety of high-quality nutrients to function correctly. Over ninety different nutrients are necessary to ensure adequate development from the time of conception until death — everything we ingest, food and chemicals, influence the growth and sustainability of our mind and body. A child's diet deficient in nutrients, in addition to inconsistent eating habits, is a high risk for cognitive impairment, obesity, and other long-term problems (Urban Child Institute, 2011). The effects of nutrient shortages depend on the extent and duration of the deficiency.

The role of nutrition is complex. Our entire body requires specific nutrients to function correctly. There is overwhelming global evidence-based research that shows how any nutrient deficiency can be detrimental to our quality of life.

In many cases, our needs change as we age. Early shortages can impair development and the ability to learn. Later in life, malnutrition can cause premature aging, dementia, and degenerative diseases.

Our brain is the ultimate command-center for the development of our body and mind; it regulates all body functions. Thereby, nutritional deficiencies that cause developmental brain dysfunction early in life may lead to physical and mental disorders that appear later in life (Liu, 2015). At all ages, nutrient deficits that affect the physiological processes of the brain cause less efficient communication between brain cells and other organs (Urban Child Institute, 2011). If our command-center gets messed up from malnutrition, it can send wrong messages to other organs that are responsible for manufacturing supplies such as enzymes, hormones, and neurotransmitters. Our brain also controls when and how those supplies get used for carrying out all the vital functions.

Paradoxically, researchers established an unexpected relationship between the mass production of cheap nutrient-deficient foods and obesity. Cheaply processed foods have become the gateway to many other health problems over the past decade. People fed high-volumes of poor-quality foods are more likely to become overweight with malnutrition, which leads to chronic illnesses, (Scheier, 2005), (Holt-Giménez, 2008).

The one thing all foods provide, regardless of its nutrient or non-nutrient value, is energy. Energy units are calories. The abbreviation for calories is Kcal. The number of calories an animal should consume daily is based on weight and activity levels. During times of growth, repair, and healing, our body may need additional high-quality calories, especially protein, to have enough energy to heal itself.

Our body stores excess energy in cells in the form of fat, but having excess energy stored in fat does not guarantee enough energy to meet the needs of your body or overcome illnesses. The quality of the calories put into storage may come back to haunt you when losing a lot of weight or during times of illness. Our stored fat is involved in several physiological functions, including metabolic regulation, energy storage, and endocrine functions. It also acts as a buffer from exposures to toxins, which during times of drastic weight loss, those toxins can be released back into the bloodstream only to cause metabolic and liver toxicity (Kim, 2011) (La Merrill M, 2013).

When food is broken down into tiny molecules, our body identifies them as either macro- or micronutrients. Macronutrients are needed in large quantities compared to micronutrients, which are needed in much smaller quantities, but all are equally vital to life. Each type of nutrient provides distinct benefits that are necessary to keep us healthy, but too much can also cause us harm.

MACRONUTRIENTS

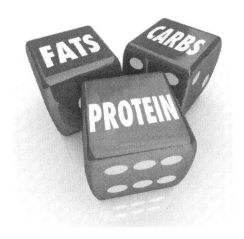

Macronutrient particles are used mainly to manufacture enzymes, hormones, and neurotransmitters. Nucleotides and proteins are responsible for encoding, replicating, transmitting, and carrying out genetic information. These internally produced chemicals support every system in our body and therefore are thought to be the most vital of macronutrients. The information within our genes is kind of like our instruction manual; there is a list of parts with instructions of what to put where and how each piece is intended to work. Too bad there isn't a troubleshooting guide included at birth!

Our body needs a constant assortment of nutrients in sufficient quantities to build supplies necessary to regularly restore, update, and replace every part of our body, including skin, blood cells, bone, and cartilage.

Some nutrients are *non-essential* because a healthy body will efficiently use protein, carbohydrate, fats, and micronutrients to manufacture these vital components. Therefore, we do not need to consume those specific nutrients in their complete form. Whereas, *essential* nutrients need to be eaten regularly because our body is not capable of manufacturing them.

There are four types of macronutrients:

1. Nucleotides bind molecules together to form *Nucleic Acids*
2. Proteins breakdown into *amino acids*
3. Carbohydrates breakdown into *sugar* and *starches*
4. Fats breakdown into *lipids* and *fatty acids*

#1: Nucleotides → Nucleic Acids

Nucleotides are the basic structural units that make up nucleic acids. Every cell of all living things is comprised of many nucleic acids, which are our genetic makeup. Therefore, they are vital to our biological welfare. Life cannot exist without nucleic acids.

Nucleic acids are semi-essential nutrients. Under normal circumstances, when a person consumes a well-balanced nutrient-rich diet, their cells absorb proteins and other nutrients that get processed into nucleic acids and are then packaged into tiny molecules, loaded into our cells. Our blood then delivers them to the rest of our body. People with poor nutrition or problems with absorbing nutrients may require additional dietary supplements to produce enough nucleic acids.

Nucleic acids create, encode, and store information inside each cell. They also translate and transmit specific information to outside the cell. There are two primary kinds of nucleic acids:

☺ Deoxyribonucleic acid (DNA): Blueprint and instructions
☺ Ribonucleic acid (RNA): Carries out the instructions

In general, our DNA and RNA are our genes. Our genes control every function inside and outside the cells of our body. They even pass our genetic information on to future generations. Our genes determine what we are at the time of conception: A plant, animal, or microbe. Additional genes control what variety of a species we become and are responsible for our unique features, such as hair and eye color, weight, height and so forth

Every trait within the makeup of all living things is packaged separately into molecules. Each trait-packet is organized in a specific order along the strands of our chromosomes. Like a manufacturing assembly line, whereas our trait-packets are like crates full of supplies that are organized in a specific order according to the order, each crate will be used. The strands of chromosomes are pairs of DNA and RNA, which contain the blueprints with instructions on how each living thing functions. These blueprints with instructions are called nucleotide sequences.

Inside each molecule, our DNA acts like an electrical wire that transfers electrons across the span of our chromosomes. Our cells take advantage of this trait to help locate and repair any mutation that can be potentially harmful to our DNA. This wire-like property of DNA is also involved in a different critical cellular function, which is replicating DNA. When cells divide and replicate themselves in our bodies, the double-stranded helix of DNA is copied. An essential protein required for replicating DNA depends on electrons traveling through DNA. "Nature is the best chemist. It knows exactly how to take advantage of DNA electron-transport chemistry" (Clavin, 2017) (O'Brien, 2017).

The arrangement of chromosomes in every living thing is a specific genetic code that regulates what we are through the replication of Vertical Gene Transfer (VGT). VTG transfers information about our two parents onto our genes. In nature, we have no control over the traits we inherit from our parents.

After birth, our genetic code is influenced by the foods we eat, the air we breathe, any chemicals we smoke, ingest or absorb, and many other environmental exposures. Where we live may have different minerals in the soil that another relative may not be exposed to, and therefore, even though you share similar DNA, your health may be very different.

When fragments of mutated DNA from nucleotides get into our cells, they can mix with our DNA and trigger changes. This is called Horizontal Gene Transfer (HGT), which we are exposed to from the environment we live in. HGT comes from our lifestyle choices, which we can control in terms of choosing what we eat, where we live, and where we work. Both VTG and HGT affect if and when we succumb to various diseases and degenerative changes as we age.

Mother Nature has equipped every living plant and animal with specific numbers of chromosomes. Within the cells of every living thing, there is a constant replication of its cells going on. During this process, our body detects any worn-out molecules that need to be repaired or replaced. Our DNA contains the entire design and instructions of our body. Our RNA unzips the pairs of DNA into two strands and then uses that information to replicate into two new strands of DNA.

Mother Nature has maintained its many different kinds of plants and animals using these DNA molecules to reproduce copies of themselves. This is what makes two humans produce another human. Humans have 46 chromosomes, which are 23 pairs of the same instructions. These are the blueprints for specific traits common to all humans, such as two arms, two legs, one trunk, and only one head. The rest of the chromosomes then determine hair and eye color and how tall we grow. Some chromosomes carry genetic defects that pass from generation to generation. The transfer of inherited traits is called Vertical Gene Transfer (VGT).

Cows have 60 chromosomes / 30 pairs. A chicken has 78 chromosomes / 39 pairs. Other forms of life have specific numbers of chromosomes that are unique to their species. When a male and female mate in nature, their chromosomes must line up to create the same specifics. If their chromosomes can't line up, then life cannot be created. In organic-nature, when two different species cross-breed, such as a horse and a donkey, their offspring is a mule. Their baby mule will always be sterile and unable to reproduce itself. Hybrid plants are either infertile or possess the genes of one of the original parent plants. Hybrid plants cannot produce offspring that are the same hybrid plant.

Mother nature limited the reproductive-mating to similar species, which safeguards the ongoing exitance of each form of life. When cells divide, carbon mixes with protein to reproduce an exact copy of the cells' chromosomes. Its replication is a genetic process that occurs during cell division. When a strand of DNA is damaged, the DNA blueprint instructs the chromosome to repair the damage or kill that cell completely.

If a defective chromosome on a strand of DNA were to survive, it could incorrectly repair itself and pass the genetic abnormality on to other cells during reproduction, (Jackson, 2002).

RNA replicates, translates, and transports the codes for the use of protein DNA. Whereas DNA contains the blueprint for life, RNA puts that information to use. Our RNA instructs enzymes and hormones to carry out specific functions. The different types of RNA include messenger, transfer, recombinant, and ribosomal RNA.

DNA does not leave the nucleus (center) of a cell; therefore, it is RNA that transports DNA signals to target locations. Under normal and healthy conditions, our DNA and RNA remain consistent by using its DNA information to replicate itself during the phase of being unzipped and duplicated. Any mutation in our nucleic acid can have dire consequences resulting in congenital disabilities, the onset of disease, weakened immune system, dysfunctional organs, and sensory malfunctions such as blindness and hearing loss.

When an environmental exposure has damaged one or more chromosomes in the DNA of any type of life, it can permanently impair all future DNA instructions in such a way as to replicate the damaged cells instead of killing them, and this replaces the original healthy instructions.

The newly created DNA will then instruct future cell replications to produce different effects that may or may not harm that body (SCHS-OSHA Alliance, 2017). Multiple studies have proven that DNA and RNA from foods containing Genetically Modified Organisms (GMO) have trans-genetic fragments that can mix with DNA during cell division and replication, causing that person or animal's DNA to mutate (GMO Awareness, 2014). If this happens, the effect may present itself quickly or manifest slowly over the decades.

Many environmental exposures, such as pesticides, genetically altered organisms, and chemicals, can damage your cells in this same manner. There is a considerable threat of mutations to your original healthy cells when your natural DNA and RNA are exposed to mutant fragments from transgenetic materials found in our foods and environmental impurities. Mutant fragments can attach to the newly formed DNA during its phase repairing and replace its worn-out cells.

A mutation is any permanent change in the number or structure of the DNA and/or RNA in a cell. Genotoxic is a general term that applies to agents or processes that alter the structure, information content, or segregation of DNA. Genotoxicity is any method that interferes with your routine DNA replication processes, or which in a non-physiological manner temporarily alter its replication, which ultimately results in new instructions telling our body to act in a way that may help or harm your health (Fang, 2014). One study demonstrated how a transplanted DNA strand interfered with the stacking mode of DNA base pairs, which caused DNA cleavage and degradation of that DNA and, ultimately, genotoxicity (Fang, 2014).

Synthetic and Transgenetic Nucleic Acids

As the Anti-Organic Movement covertly strives to replace organic foods with POB, the third type of nucleic acid has risen to enormous proportions in the foods sold to American consumers. GMO foods and chemical additives that contain mutations do not occur naturally; they are a manufactured commodity made by food scientists and engineers (NIH, 2016).

Scientists have the technology and unlimited support of lawmakers to alter natural traits in organic plants, animals, and microorganisms by removing or adding chains of molecules along a strand of DNA or RNA. By transplanting genes from different forms of life into another, they can create unique plants and animals that have traits not typically found in natural plants or animals. Food engineers have the ability to implant chains of artificial nucleic acids, which are known as 'free or naked DNA,' into our food without our knowledge.

Original, during the 1990s, when genetically modifying food was first deregulated, scientists made viruses from fragments of genes and injected those virus fragments into the DNA of plants and animals to change the natural traits of those recipients. In more recent years, the discoveries of two currently emerging technologies are, the gene-editing tool CRISPR and lab-grown meat from cultures. CRISPR allows food engineers to change the DNA of any organism with greater precision easily. Its founder envisioned its use for 'treating diseases, creating tastier produce and making drought-resistant crops, but she's also feared that someone might use it in secret to mess with human DNA (Brodwin E. C., 2019).

This is a real threat to the national safety of any government regulated by officials who are willing to pass legislation for unregulated voluntary food labeling (114 Congress , 2015) (110th Congress, 2008). What guarantees do consumers have that food sold to one community may contain genes that increase nutrient content, while the same food sold in another district may have harmful genes that cause infertility, diseases, or chronic illnesses to support it's $4 trillion medical industry?

The POB food industry touts that Lab-grown meat can free up meat producers from being dependent on farms by allowing for real chicken and beef to be made in a lab from animal cells instead of from slaughter. Two such companies already selling meats using these technologies claim that technologies like CRISPR allow them to safely increase the quality of their cell growth to make the meat tastier, healthier, and more sustainable than slaughtered meat.

Their first prototypes cost $18,000 a pound, putting the price-tag of a clean quarter-pounder at roughly the same cost as monthly rent for an average 2-bedroom apartment in San Francisco. However, in two years, the company was able to reduce the price to $2,400 per pound.

Similarly, the first prototype cost per sausage-link was $2500 but has been lowered to only $250 per link. By feeding their cells with a nutrient-dense mixture of fetal bovine serum (FBS) made from the blood of pregnant slaughtered cows, these two food companies are producing lab-made meats, (Brodwin E. , 2019). The problem is, these POB food industrialists are using organic resources to make unaffordable lab-made meats that are not regulated or require any testing for safety. Just because your cuisine tastes great, does not guarantee it is safe to eat; if there are additives that have the potential to unknowingly cause infertility or illness to a specific social group, race, or religion, it is not safe to consume that will cause preventable medical conditions that are expensive to treat.

The most significant consequence of breaking DNA strands to transplant into foreign species are its mutations and genomic-instability that cause neurological dysfunctions, infertility, and many diseases including a variety of cancers such as skin, colon, breast, and prostate, (Cell Biolabs Inc., 2019):

Oxidative DNA damage refers to the oxidation of specific bases that are the most common marker for oxidative DNA damage and can be measured in virtually any species. It is formed and enhanced most often by chemical carcinogens. Similar oxidative damage can occur in RNA, which has been implicated in various neurological disorders.

Hydrolytic DNA damage involves the total removal of individual bases, which can be particularly mutagenic when left unrepaired because they can inhibit transcription. Hydrolytic DNA damage may result from the biochemical reactions of various metabolites.

Various types of radiation can damage DNA in the form of DNA strand breaks. This involves a cut in one or both DNA strands; double-strand breaks are especially dangerous and can be mutagenic since they can potentially affect the expression of multiple genes.

By adding, removing, and exchanging the sequence of DNA in living things, scientists can add or remove traits that mother nature had not intended. For example, in 2007, the FDA approved goat editing to produce anti-clotting milk and insulin grown from bacteria (Greenwood, 2018). Since then, scientists have begun to add strands of human genes to pigs to make them grow human organs to be surgically transplanted into humans (Lerner, 2017) (Weintraub, 2017).

There are many evidence-based-research warning that naked DNA survives in the digestive system, which can merge into our own DNA during cell replication, causing dysfunction to our organs, diseases, and weakening our immune system (Ho, 1999). In other words, anyone who consumes GMO foods may be exposed to naked DNA that can be absorbed into our cells. Once in our cells, the free DNA can match-up with our chromosomes during its DNA and RNA cell division. If this occurs, the cell's entire messaging system and DNA instructions can be changed. This is called Horizontal Gene Transformation (HGT) (Lerner, A., 2017).

Long ago, the National Institute of Health (NIH) created guidelines to protect the food-industries scientists and food engineers from the dangers related to the research of artificial nucleic acid. These guidelines are their Laboratory Safety Monograph, which has not changed since its creation in 1979; Section IV-B-1-i. specifically warns, ' Certain medical conditions may place a laboratory worker at increased risk in any endeavor where infectious agents are handled. Any laboratory workers with gastrointestinal disorders or prescribed treatments with steroids, immunosuppressive drugs, or antibiotics should not engage in research with potentially hazardous organisms during their treatment or illness' (Barkley, 1979).

In 2007, The 110th Congress amended the FDA and Federal Meat Inspection Act to forbid organic meat competitors from labeling their animals products as cloned-free, "unless it also includes a statement indicating that a food that does not contain cloned meat has no bearing on the safety of the food for human consumption," (110th Congress, 2008).

In 1998 the UK Ministry of Agriculture, Fisheries, and Food (MAFF) notified the US Food and Drug Administration (FDA) of the following warnings,' (Ho, 1999):

Transgenic DNA can spread to farmworkers and food processors via dust and pollen.

Antibiotic-resistant genes may spread to bacteria in the mouth, as the mouth contains bacteria that readily take up and incorporate foreign DNA. Similar transformable bacteria are present in the respiratory tracts.

Antibiotic-resistant genes may spread to bacteria in the environment, which then serves as a reservoir for antibiotic resistance genes.

DNA is not readily degraded during food processing, nor in the silage, hence transgenic DNA can spread to animals in animal feed.

Foreign DNA can be delivered into mammalian cells by bacteria that can enter into the cells

The ampicillin resistance gene in the transgenic maize undergoing 'farm-scale' field-trials in the UK and elsewhere is very mutable and may compromise treatment for meningitis and other bacterial infections, should the gene be transferred horizontally to the bacteria. The potential hazards of horizontal gene transfer are unlike those we have ever experienced.

There are many factors in our lifestyles that may dynamically impact our DNA and RNA. Conditions in our digestive system can make us vulnerable to naked nucleic acids created by the POB food industry. Nucleic acids can be taken up by our cells to multiply, mutate and recombine indefinitely" (Ho, 1999).

Rebekah S. Mead

#2: Proteins → Amino Acids

Our digestive system breaks down proteins into many different kinds of tiny nutrient-particles called amino acids. Like all other nutrients, the usable amino acids get extracted, filtered, and packaged into our cells to be shipped to organs where they will be assembled into products our body uses. The restructured amino acids are used to make nucleic acids, fat, energy, hormones, enzymes, neurotransmitters, and many other life-sustaining supplies. While in the form of amino acids, they reside in all of our cells in the form of building blocks. They provide most of our cell's structure while helping each cell to carry out its own functions.

Our body does not store protein in the form of amino acids that can be accessed whenever needed. Any excess protein consumed in a day is converted into fat and stored as fat, even though our need for protein is constant throughout our life. Therefore, the human body needs to consume moderate amounts of high-quality protein every day and increase protein during times of growth and healing.

Amino acids are so essential to the developing body during childhood that any deficiency can set the stage for degenerative and psychological disorders later in life. For example, the amino acid tyrosine is one of the building blocks needed to make dopamine and norepinephrine, while another amino acid known as tryptophan is used to manufacture serotonin, all of which support our mental and physical neurological functions. A child's diet that is deficient in these proteins can trigger many health complications that may not appear until years or decades later, (Khan. A., 2017).

Swiss Researchers found a deficiency of brain chemicals were triggered by low levels of specific amino acids that led to a chain reaction of other amino acid deficiencies; "children with ADHD appear to have nearly 50 percent lower levels of an amino acid called tryptophan, a protein which helps in the production of dopamine, noradrenaline, and serotonin. It also is important for attention and learning" (Collingwood, 2018). A decrease in dopamine activity reduces the transmission of messages throughout the body sent by the neurotransmitter system (Johansson, 2011).

Our body is continuously building and restoring itself, whereas protein is the primary nutrient responsible for repairing and healing our body. It also plays an essential role in its own digestion and distribution. If there is ever a shortage of consumed fats or carbohydrates, proteins come to our rescue by getting converted into fat for energy (Majda, 2014), but this can take away from protein being used to perform its many valuable functions and lead to protein deficiencies.

It is essential to our health that high-quality protein be consumed daily. "Protein quality depends not only on the amino acid composition but also on protein bioavailability or digestibility, (Arendt, 2013). Causes of protein deficiency are:

☺ Poor bioavailability: A protein source is not easily absorbed & used, or a person is allergic, causing rejection
☺ Low-quality proteins: Made from inferior products that produce inferior amino acids
☹ No protein: Foods that have no protein

As vital chemically-reactive building blocks, their quality is at least as important as the number of proteins consumed. Poor quality and /or insufficient amounts of any amino acids can cause many health problems, including, (Collingwood, 2018) (Behar, 2016), (Fulgoni, 2008), (Khan. A., 2017), (Sloan, 2007):

☹ Heart diseases
☹ Impaired mental health: Depression, anxiety, restlessness, tension, sorrow, and crankiness
☹ Anger, impulsiveness and violent tendencies
☹ Attention Deficient Hyperactivity Disorder (ADHA), autism, schizophrenia, and bipolar disorder
☹ Kwashiorkor: Malnutrition causing swollen belly and limbs, skin disorders, poor muscle formation and hinders mental and physical development in children
☹ Marasmus: Protein inadequacy that triggers muscle weakness and makes sufferers more prone to infections
☺ Edema: Undermines fluid balance by triggering swelling that can cause:
   o Harm to arms and legs
   o Stains to our skin
   o Hypertension
   o Stiff joints
☹ Organ failure: For example, kidney failure when the body cannot eliminate waste
☺ Weak immune system
☹ Poor wound healing

☺ Hair loss
☺ Leptin & Insulin Resistance
☺ Neurological disorders
☺ Hormone imbalance: Infertility, erectile dysfunction
☺ Pre-mature aging and degenerative diseases

Protein comes from the foods we eat: Poultry, seafood, dairy, eggs, produce, nuts, and grains. Once ingested, it breaks down into twenty-two kinds of amino acids that are either:
☺ Non-essential
☺ Essential
☺ Semi-essential

Non-essential amino acids are internally manufactured using other substances to create the amounts needed and, therefore, do not need to be individually consumed. They are synthesized from carbohydrates and other amino acids.

Those we cannot produce and, therefore, must come from the proteins we consume are essential amino acids. *Essential amino acids* are (Owens, 1999):

☺ *Phenylalanine:*
  o Crucial in the production of other amino acids
  o Effects skin, mood, and tolerance to pain
☺ *Valine:*
  o Promotes healthy growth, repair tissues & aids in muscle recovery
  o Regulate blood sugar
  o Provides the body with energy
  o Stimulates the central nervous system and is needed for proper mental functioning
☺ *Threonine:*
  o Makes up elastin, collagen, and enamel protein
  o Promotes proper fat metabolism in the liver
  o Aids metabolism throughout the GI tract
☺ *Tryptophan:*
  o Helps the body make specialized amino acids
  o Aids in the absorption of vitamins
  o Is needed to make brain chemicals
☺ *Isoleucine:*

- o Broken-down to extract energy from muscle tissue
- o Helps repair and restore muscles
- ☺ *Methionine:*
  - o Needed for the production of immune cells and the development of nerve function
  - o It is an antioxidant that plays a significant role in the liver's repair and rebuilding processes
- ☺ *Leucine:*
  - o Metabolism of proteins
  - o Regulates blood sugar levels
  - o Promotes growth and the recovery of muscle and bone tissues
  - o Aids in the production of the growth hormone
- ☺ *Lysine:*
  - o Vital for proper growth; plays many important roles:
    - Manufacturing of carnitine, which transforms fatty acids into energy and lowers cholesterol levels
    - Helps absorb calcium, which is needed for bone health
    - Manufacturing collagen, which is required for building connective tissues such as tendons, cartilage, and skin
    - Helps process fats into energy and lower cholesterol

Semi-essential amino acids come from amino acids that most adults produce enough of, but children cannot. Therefore, it is essential for children to get these amino acids from the protein they consume daily:

- ☺ *Arginine:*
  - o Is extremely important to bodies under stress, for instance:
    - During childhood when children are rapidly growing
    - Patients with burns, sepsis, kidney disease, liver failure, intestinal disorders, and other trauma that requires healing
    - Proteins rich in arginine are essential for the development and maintenance of the immune system especially in children and people with illnesses and injuries (Babineau, 1994)
  - o Relaxes blood vessels
  - o Aids in the metabolism of proteins

☺ *L-Cysteine:*
  o It is vital for the synthesis of amino acids and other nutrients. It creates stiffness and stability in connective tissues. A deficiency affects aging in terms of degenerative changes such as neurological disorders, liver disease, and malabsorption disorders. L-cysteine is responsible for (Aminoacidstudies.org, unk), (Immunehealthscience.com, 2018):
      • Highly detoxifying; an anti-oxidative and anti-aging nutrient that attacks free radicals that can cause degrative changes
      • Strengthens our immunity by fueling our macrophages, which are our killer cells that attack infections
      • Inhibits inflammation
  o Manufactures structural proteins in our connective tissue which aids in the health of nerves, tendons, bones, hair, and skin
  o Necessary for conducting electrical nervous impulses
  o Supports the digestive and vascular systems
  o Promotes male fertility

☺ *Histidine:*
  o Is vital in the regulation of gene expression by inhibiting or activating DNA and RNA
  o Required for growth and tissue repair and blood cell production
  o Needed for the creation of the neurotransmitter histamine
  o Protect tissues from damage caused by radiation or heavy metals
  o Plays a significant role in obesity and metabolic syndrome
  o Relaxes blood vessels which help the flow
  o A person weighing 154 pounds should consume around 700mg of histidine per day (Whitbread, 2018)

Nucleic acids and protein are vital to our genetic makeup. Whereas, protein and fat provide satiety that makes us feel full when enough nutrients have been consumed to meet all of our bodily functions. An increase in dietary protein from 15% to 30% of all calories consumed can increase our leptin sensitivity. This can result in a natural and healthy weight loss (Weigle D, 2005). Unlike fat, protein is only 4 calories per gram. Because it is vital to so many functions, daily intake of calories from protein should be between 20% to 30% of the total calories consumed. During times of growth, illness, or injury, it should be 30% to 35% of all calories consumed.

The way to calculate the percentage of protein consumed is to:

a. Identify the total number of calories you consume daily
b. Multiple the desired percentage times total calories, which will equal the total number of calories from protein. *Total Calories x percentage = # of calories from protein*
c. Divide that number by 4 protein calories per gram. This will equal how many grams of protein you should consume. *# of calories from protein ÷ 4 = grams of protein daily*
d. Divide the total number of grams by 30, and this will tell you how many ounces of protein you should consume daily. *# grams ÷ 30 = how many ounces daily*

For example, a diet of 2000 calories daily with a goal of 20% protein and 30% protein:

[2000 x .20 = 400] ÷ 4 calories = 100 grams of protein daily (about 3.5 ounces)

[2000 x .30 = 600] ÷ 4 calories = 150 grams of protein daily (about 5 ounces)

Since foods containing protein also contain other nutrients, usually calories can be applied to other recommended daily nutrients. In other words, nutrient-rich foods contain a variety of nutrients in each calorie. For example, a slice of organic beef weighing 90 grams (3 ounces) provides both protein and fat.

Be aware that not all protein is created equal. "Dietary proteins are divided into two kinds of proteins: complete proteins, which include all essential amino acids in the exact amounts required by the body for growth and incomplete proteins, which are deficient in one or more essential amino acids" (Behar, 2016).

Many Americans are not consuming enough, high-quality protein (Fulgoni, 2008). The quality of what we consume is at least as important as the quantity. Poor quality protein breaks down into inferior quality amino acids that are then used to build poor quality nucleic acids and other life-sustaining chemicals. The difference can be as drastic as using straw versus slate to construct the roof of your house.

Strength and durability rely on the quality of the materials used. Protein comes from many sources. Organic sources are consistent in their nutrients, whereas nutrients of non-organic, trans-genetic, and GMO sources depend on what genes have been added and/or removed and how well the recipient incorporates those genes into its own DNA.

Due to unpredictability and the wide variations of Non-Organic foods, I only listed the protein values of organic sources.

Organic Meat (Beef, Pork) Protein
- ☺ Meat protein is complete; it contains all the essential amino acids.
- ☺ Low in allergies
- ☺ 100% 4 oz. beef has about 240 calories, 23 grams of protein and 20 grams of fat; 93% fat-free 4 oz burger is about 170 calories with 23 grams of protein and 9 grams of fat, (Sparkpeople, 2013)
- ☺ 100% 4 oz lean Pork-Loin with fat removed has about 173 calories with 26 grams of protein and only 6 grams of fat. Ground pork and sausage, on the other hand, may have more fat than protein, for instance, 4 oz ground pork is about 298 calories with 19 grams of protein and 24 grams of fat, (Sparkpeople, 2013)
- ☺ Depending on the cut and how much fat is used to make sausage or ground pork, some pork can be nutrient-dense, while lean cuts can be very nutrient-rich with low calories.
- ☺ It is a dependable and excellent source of protein and has many micronutrients

Organic Poultry Protein
- ☺ Cage-free poultry roam free and consume natural insects and non-GMO plants, grains
- ☺ Usually less expensive than meat
- ☺ Nutrient-rich: High in protein with less fat than beef.
- ☺ A 4 oz serving of chicken is about 31 grams of protein with about 8 grams of fat

Wild Caught Fish and Seafood
- ☺ High in protein and low in fat, per 4 oz serving broiled, (Superior Fish Company):
  - o Haddock: 120 calories with 26 grams of protein and 1.3 grams of fat
  - o Lobster: 160 cal. with 26 grams of protein and 1 gram of fat

o Sockeye Alaskan Salmon: 150 cal. with 32 grams of protein and 14 grams of fat
o Tuna, Yellowfin: 160 cal. with 33 grams of protein and 1.3 grams fat

☺ Nutrient-rich: High in protein and low in calories and fat
☹ High in allergies
☹ Poly-Chlorinated Biphenyls (PCB) contaminated fish, according to EPA, can cause birth defects, neurological disorders, and cancer. PCB's were banned in 1977, but continue to contaminate the ocean, freshwater, land, and air, (WDHS, 2018), (WDF, Unk.)

Organic Eggs

☺ Whole eggs are nutrient-dense with high bioavailability amino acid profile than egg whites; egg yolks contain all of the vitamins, minerals, antioxidants, and Omega-3 fatty acids
☺ High in protein and fat: 4 ounces of eggs are about 164 calories with 15 grams of protein and 11 grams of fat. One large egg is about 72 calories with 6 grams of protein and 5 grams of fat
☺ Contains vitamins A, B12, D and E
☺ Contains minerals: magnesium, phosphorus, and potassium
☹ High in allergies
☺ Aside from protein, egg whites have no nutrient value

Organic Milk & Dairy

☺ Has many applications: Drink, add to cereal and coffee, used to make ice cream, butter, yogurt, cheese and in baked goods
☺ 8 oz of 100% milk has about 160 calories with 9 grams of protein and 9 grams of fat
☺ 8 oz of 1% low-fat milk has 120 calories with 10 grams of protein and 2.5 grams of fat

Organic Whey, (Eat This Much Inc, 2019), (USDA, 2015)

☺ One tablespoon is about 55 calories with 10 gm protein and < 1 gm fat
☺ Whey protein concentrate (WPC) is a family of dry dairy ingredients used to add concentrated whey protein to food products, (USAID.Gov, 2016)
☺ A byproduct of cheese during its manufacturing. Organic whey is a rich source of protein made from the remaining liquid after milk is curdled and strained.

☺ When produced from organic animals, it is a complete protein which consists of all nine essential amino acids essential for protein synthesis

☹ The way whey is packaged, it may be chemically treated and adulterated therefore losing its nutritional properties (Cuff, 2013)

☹ Processed whey removes fats and carbohydrates in addition to some of the protein. The end product may have 34% to 80% of protein, depending on how it's processed, (USAID.Gov, 2016). If it's processed with heat, the proteins can be denatured (not good), (Cuff, 2013)

☹ Whey from animals fed GMO grains may contain some of those contaminants

☹ High in allergies

☹ Higher cholesterol content

Organic Grain, (Norwitz, 2007)

☺ Good source of bioavailable protein and healthy fat

☺ Various types of grain protein. For example, a few common ones are:

- o Amaranthaceae: Amaranth
- o Chenopodiaceae: Oats
- o Gluten (Triticeae): Wheat, barley, rye
- o Poaceae: Wheat, barley, rye, millet, buckwheat, corn starch, white & wild rice
- o Polygonaceae: Buckwheat

☺ Per 4 oz cup of pure grains:

- o Amaranthaceous is about 87 Kcal, 14 gms protein, and 7 gms fat
- o Oats are about 78 Kcal with 13 grams of protein and 11 grams of fat; binds with cholesterol and helps to reduce LDL
- o Barley is about 74 Kcal with 8 gm protein and 1gm fat
- o Wheat is about 84 Kcal, with 15 gms protein and 35 gms fat; gives elasticity to baked goods
- o Buckwheat is about 60 Kcal with 8 gms protein and 4 gms fat

#3: Carbohydrates → Starch and Sugar

Carbohydrates are the sugars, starches, and fibers found in fruits, grains, vegetables, and milk products. Each kind of carbohydrate performs distinct jobs in the body.

Fiber is an essential nutrient that aids digestion:
- ☺ It does not get broken-down or absorbed
- ☺ Dietary fiber is commonly known as roughage or bulk
- ☺ It comes from parts of plants our body can't digest; instead, it passes through our stomach, small intestine, and colon.
- ☺ In the large intestines, it stimulates activity in our microbiome (gut flora) that maintains and restores our gut back to a healthy status.
- ☺ There are two types of fiber:
  - o *Soluble fiber*
    - Dissolves in water to form a gel-like material
    - Binds to cholesterol which lowers the LDL circulating in the blood
    - Aids in regulating glucose levels
    - Is found in oats, peas, beans, apples, citrus fruits, carrots, and barley
  - o *Insoluble fiber*
    - Promotes the movement of material through your digestive system
    - Increases stool bulk that prevents constipation
    - Is found in whole-wheat flour, wheat bran, nuts, beans and vegetables, such as cauliflower, green beans, and potatoes
    - This is the fiber that helps restore gut flora

Dietary fiber found in whole fresh fruits, vegetables, and entire grains stimulates peristalsis and flushes out fats and waste. Drinking plenty of fluids keeps stools soft and easy to pass. Yogurt and other probiotic foods contain live bacterial cultures that promote healthy microbiota but be aware of any food additives or chemicals that may inhibit the benefits.

Fiber is a complex carbohydrate with many benefits to your health:
- ☺ It slows down the digestion process and prevents sugar from forming too quickly. This helps the body maintain blood sugars levels, so they will not spike.
- ☺ Provides nutrition for our microbiota
- ☺ Increases bulk of stool to aid in its elimination

Starch is a complex carbohydrate:
- ☺ It is slowly digested by the body and becomes blood glucose that is absorbed into the bloodstream to be used as energy
- ☺ It is the primary dietary source of carbohydrates for the body

Sugar is a simple carbohydrate:
- ☺ It is the basic building block of molecules for every type of carbohydrate
- ☺ Unlike fiber and starch, it breaks down quickly and easily into glucose which is used by the body as a primary energy source

The recommended daily amount (RDA) of carbohydrates is 45% and 65% of total calories consumed. One gram of carbs equals 4 calories: 30 grams is equal to about 1 ounce, multiplied by 4 calories equals about 120 calories per ounce of carbs. Using the same formula as we did for proteins because the number of calories in carbs and protein are the same per gram:

- ❖ A diet of 2000 calories per day, of which 45% to 60% comes from carbs, would equal 900 to 1200 calories from carbohydrates. Divided by 4 Kcal. equates to 225 to 300 grams or 7.5 to 10 ounces of carbohydrates daily.

The right carbohydrates are very beneficial to our health. They help:

- ☺ Brain function: Influence mood, behavior, and motivation
- ☺ Neuromuscular ability to transmit signals
- ☺ Energy levels: Quick, reliable energy source
- ☺ Central nervous system function
- ☺ Energy Storage: Prevents protein from being used as an energy source
- ☺ Metabolism: Enables Breakdown of fat into fatty acids
- ☺ Healthy microbiota (gut flora) in large intestines fight disease
- ☺ The lining of our intestines and bowel movements (elimination of waste)

When it comes to nutrition, not all carbohydrates are created equal. Carbohydrates are classified as simple or complex. The difference between the two forms is the chemical structure which affects how quickly the sugar in these carbohydrates get digested and used for energy. Generally speaking, simple carbs are already in digested form and ready to be used as instant energy. Complex carbs utilize the entire digestive system to break it down, sort it out, filter and distribute it in the most beneficial ways. It is the process of digestion that keeps us strong and healthy.

When any part of digestion is bypassed, imbalances are likely to occur. For instance, too many simple carbs consumed at one feeding will bypass the liver and go directly to the pancreas. Any overload of excessive unfiltered calories can overwhelm and confuse the pancreas, so it converts most of the contents into fat to be stored immediately. In small amounts, natural, simple sugars are a source for quick energy, but too much over a long period of time can deplete the hormones leptin and insulin, causing leptin and/or insulin resistance.

Simple carbohydrates made with processed and refined sugars are found in candy, soda, syrups, and beer. These processed foods remove natural starches and fibers found in carbohydrates and also remove its natural fat and proteins. They replace those vital nutrients with simple carbohydrates used to restore its texture and taste. These simple carbs do not contain vitamins, minerals, or fiber. Replacing saturated fats with simple carbs increases our risk of heart disease, high LDL cholesterol, and type 2 diabetes (Szalay, 2017).

Types of carbohydrates are:
- ☺ Simple Carbs:
  - o Monosaccharides contain one sugar molecule. These are the most basic carbs that cannot be broken down any further. They are fruit (fructose), milk (galactose) or a combination of both
  - o Disaccharides contain two sugar molecules. These are sucrose (table sugar), lactose (from dairy) and maltose (found in beer and some vegetables)
- ☺ Complex carbohydrates:
  - o Are called polysaccharides because have three or more sugars
  - o They are often referred to as starchy foods. These include beans, peas, lentils, legumes, nuts, potatoes, corn, parsnips, whole-grain breads, and cereals

When glucose is not immediately used for energy, the body can store up to 2,000 calories in the liver and skeletal muscles in the form of glycogen. Once glycogen stores are full, carbs are converted and stored as fat. When there is insufficient carbohydrate intake or stores, the body will start to convert protein into fuel. This can be especially problematic during times of healing because protein builds and restores tissues while carbs provide the energy. Using protein instead of carbohydrates for fuel then puts unnecessary stress on the kidneys because the byproducts of protein used for fuel are then filtered in the kidneys and eliminated in our urine.

Carbohydrates also greatly influence how efficiently and accurately our neurotransmitters send instructions to organs. Poor quality and imitation foods, food additives, and chemicals that inhibit signal or over-excite its transmission can cause neuromuscular diseases, such as Parkinson's disease. One military study observed how carbohydrate's influence neurotransmitter's in special populations, such as individuals who develop unusual symptoms in response to foods or specific nutrients. One example found people who craved and consumed large amounts of carbohydrate-rich snacks derived temporary relief from depressive symptoms (Wurtman, 1994).

Numerous research studies identified the importance of complex carbohydrates in the diet. The timing of carb intake throughout the day is as likely to be as important as the quality and quantity. One study noticed children fed a high protein with low complex-carbohydrate breakfast not only performed better in the classroom but were more likely to share and be kind to fellow students compared to a breakfast high in carbs with low protein, in which those children were less inclined to share.

Studies show that carbs improve neuro-transmission. A group of overweight women who cut carbs entirely from their diets for one-week then experienced problems with learning new skills and retaining general information. Another researcher showed how carbohydrates affect mental well-being. People on a high-fat - low-carb diet experienced more anxiety, frustration, depression, and anger than people on a low-fat, high-carb diet. These scientists suspect that complex carbohydrates help with the production of serotonin in the brain, which increases feelings of happiness and improves memory and recall.

In the right balance spread throughout the day, carbohydrates provide sustained energy, a robust immune system, improved neuro-signaling, and weight control. The Omniheart Randomized study revealed a diet rich in natural complex carbs increases HDL (healthy housekeepers) and lower triglycerides. By replacing bad carbs with good ones, many participants in the study improved their cholesterol numbers (Appel, 2005).

Good carbs vs. bad carbs

According to the Pritikin Longevity Center (Killoran, 1992):
☺ Good carbs are:
  o Low or moderate in calories
  o High in nutrients
  o Contain no refined sugars and refined grains
  o Are naturally high in fiber
  o Low in sodium
  o Low in saturated fat
  o Very low or have no cholesterol and trans fats

☹ Bad carbs are:
  o High in calories
  o Full of refined sugars, like High Fructose Corn Syrup, Corn Syrup, white sugar and honey
  o High in refined grains like processed white flour
  o Low in nutrients
  o Low in fiber
  o High in sodium
  o High in saturated fat
  o High in cholesterol and trans fats

#4: Fats → Lipids & Fatty Acids

Fats are one of the four primary macronutrients that are vital to life. It is a semi-essential nutrient because our body can usually produce enough from the fats, proteins, and carbohydrates we consume. Ideally, one-third of all consumed calories should come from consuming healthy fat.

Under most circumstances, there is enough fat in the American diet to meet our daily needs. Many plant and animal products contain fat in addition to other nutrients, making added fats unnecessary, but if a diet is deficient on fat, a portion or all of the protein consumed that day may be converted into fat. Therefore, people who continually consume a no-fat diet are at risk for both protein and fat-soluble vitamin deficiencies.

Fats are higher in calories than the other macronutrients, which makes them convert more readily into energy. They have nine calories per gram compared to the other macronutrients that have only four calories per gram. Therefore, our body needs only a small amount of healthy fat daily to function properly and still make up one-third of all consumed calories. The benefits of natural / organic fats are, they:

☺ Protect and insulate each body organ and the entire body
☺ Aid in the production of appetite-regulating hormones
☺ Make us feel satisfied and full
☺ Give us immediate energy
☺ Break-down, absorb and use fat-soluble vitamins
☺ Break-down, absorb and utilize minerals
☺ Help production and use of reproductive and growth hormones
☺ Provide Anti-inflammatory actions
☺ Provide energizing fuel to our immune system
☺ Provide energy

Fats are a group of chemical compounds that get broken down into fatty acids. Fatty acids are then used to make internal chemicals. There are three main types of "natural" fatty acids:

☺ Saturated
☺ Monounsaturated
☺ Polyunsaturated

Saturated fats are mostly found in animal products, whereas monounsaturated and polyunsaturated are primarily found in plants. All fatty acids are molecules composed mostly of carbon and hydrogen atoms. A saturated fatty acid has multiple hydrogen atoms attached to each carbon atom inside its molecules. Thereby, the carbons in those fats are saturated with hydrogen atoms.

Some fatty acids are missing one or more pairs of hydrogen atoms inside their molecules. This results in a gap known as "unsaturation." The fats missing one-pair of hydrogens are a monosaturated fatty acid because it has one gap. Polyunsaturated fatty acids have multiple gaps because they are missing multiple pairs of hydrogen atoms" (Infoplease, 2018).

Saturated fats

☺ Only come from animal products: Fatty meat, chicken skin, dairy and eggs

☺ At room temperature, they are usually solid, but when heated they melt

☹ In natural forms, they are a rich source of many essential nutrients that should be consumed in moderation. The AHA recommends saturated fats be less than 10% of daily calories because in large quantities they can build-up in vessels causing blockages

☺ Consuming whole milk dairy products in moderation provides health benefits, especially for children, teenagers, and elderly:
  o Improved bone health
  o Improves heart health
  o Lowers blood pressure
  o Helps regulate insulin
  o Improves mood

Lean cuts of meat and chicken are a healthier choice of saturated fat because they are also high in protein which is essential for building and restoring healthy tissue

Monounsaturated fats:

☺ Are found in plants and some fish
☺ Help reduce LDL in the blood
☺ Are usually in liquid form at room temperature
☺ Should make up 20% to 30% of daily consumed calories
☺ A seven-country study during the 1960s revealed that people in Greece and other parts of the Mediterranean region have a low rate of heart disease despite a high-fat diet that is high in monosaturated fats (Harvard Medical School, 2015).

Polyunsaturated fats:

☺ Are found in plants and fish
☺ Are usually liquid at room temperature
☺ Should make-up 20% to 30% of daily consumed calories
☺ Eating polyunsaturated fats in place of saturated fats or highly refined carbohydrates reduces LDL and triglyceride cholesterol and increases HDL
☺ Good sources (omega-3 fatty acids) are oily fish such as wild-caught salmon, mackerel, and sardines, flaxseeds, walnuts, canola oil, and un-hydrogenated (non-GMO) soybean oil. Omega-3 fatty acids:

o Help prevent and reverse heart disease and strokes.
o Reduce neurological disorders.
o Prevent dementia
o Improve learning and attention; prevents Attention Deficient Hyperactivity Disorder (ADHD).
o Reduce the need for corticosteroid medications in people with rheumatoid arthritis.
o Foods rich in Omega-6 fatty acids include non-GMO vegetable oils such as safflower, soybean, sunflower, walnut, and corn oils. Omega-6 fatty acids also protect against heart disease and strokes

Trans-fats

Not all fats were created equal. Over the last half-century, new man-made fats were created by manipulating the hydrogens. Other fats new to the food marker are the byproduct of genetically altered plants and animals. In addition to the natural fats, the food industry added Trans-fats (FDA, 2018) (Mercola, 2019) (Harvard Medical School, 2015):

☺ Industrial-made partially hydrated fats were created to prevent spoilage, maintain a solid form at room temperatures and increase texture and appearance

☺ Added to American foods since the 1950s

☺ Are in hardened vegetable fats, margarine, snack food, baked foods, processed foods, and fried foods

☺ Manufacturers use them because they do not go rancid as quickly as natural fats. Therefore, they substantially extend the shelf life of many products

☺ Have no nutritional value or benefits. The chemical reaction that makes natural fats perform the benefits listed in this section does not occur in trans-fats. Manufacturers purposely remove trans-fats' ability to Breakdown and use its chemical activities to prevent their product from rancidity, which consequently prevents any benefits from consumption

☺ Increases buildup of poor quality Low-Density Lipids (LDL) in arteries, which can result in a heart attack or stroke

☺ They are used by many fast-food restaurants

☹ Added to many low and no fat foods to replace real fat:
   o Listed as "partially hydrogenated oil" in ingredients on a label
   o If the Nutrition Facts says, their product has "0 g trans-fat," that doesn't necessarily mean it has no trans fats. It could have up to half a gram (0.5) of trans fats per serving to be listed as 0% as per USA food laws. For example, a serving size on 10 potato chips may have only 0.5 grams of trans-fat, qualifying it to be listed as 0 trans-fats, but consuming an entire bag that has 3.5 servings may have up to 1.75 grams of trans-fat which is 0.06 oz

☺ Increases overall LDL and triglycerides and reduces the HDL cholesterol

☺ It creates inflammation linked to heart disease and stroke. "For every 2% of calories from trans-fat consumed daily, the risk of heart disease rises by 23%" (Harvard Medical School, 2015)
☺ Cause obesity, diabetes, and leptin resistance
☺ Cause fat-soluble vitamin deficiencies
☺ The World Health Organization (WHO):
  o Estimates that every year, trans fat intake causes more than 500,000 deaths from cardiovascular disease
  o In 2003, recommended that trans fats make up no more than 1% of a person's diet
  o In 2018, it introduced a 6-step guide to eliminate industrially-produced trans-fatty acids from the global food supply.
☺ The American Heart Association (AHA) recommends no more than 1% of all fat consumption come from trans-fats: [(2000 x .01) ÷ 9] ÷ 2.2 = 0.075 oz
☺ In 2015 the FDA removed trans-fat from the GRAS category. By 2020, FDA mandates trans fats be removed from all foods sold in the USA (FDA, 2018)

For our body to function properly and have enough energy to meet its needs, one-third of calories consumed should come from healthy organic fats. For instance:

❖ A diet of 2000 calories, of which 33% comes from fat, would equal 660 calories from fat. Divided by 9 calories per gram equals about 73 grams of fat or about two and a half ounces of fat daily. [(2000 x .33) ÷ 9] ÷ 30 = 2.5 oz.; which is 2 Tbsp of butter plus 3 Tbsp of olive oil per day, (Convert-to.com, 2019), (Calculateme.com, 2019).

❖ A diet of 1200 calories, of which only 20% comes from fat, would equal 240 calories divided by 9 calories per gram equals about 27 grams of fat or about 0.9 ounces of fat per day. [(1200 x .20) ÷ 9] ÷ 30 = 0.9 oz.; which is one tsp of olive oil per day, (Convert-to.com, 2019)

If dieting, no less than 20% of calories should come from fats. This is to prevent health problems, but even consuming enough fat in our diet is no guarantee we are using it effectively. Like protein, not all fats are created equal. Animal sources of fat are most readily available to the body compared with plant sources. For example, omega-3 fats from plants need to be converted from a short-chain structure to a long chain to receive the health benefits from these specific fats. This conversion takes specific nutrients and enzymes, so if one is deficient in any of these supplies, this conversion may not take place. Diet, smoking, alcohol, caffeine, and stress in all its forms are a few lifestyle choices that impede the body's ability to utilize fat effectively, which can then deplete the body of co-factors that further impair our ability to use the fat we consume (Hernandez, 2019).

There are many severe consequences of not consuming enough fat. Aside from low energy and vitality, a deficiency in healthy bioavailable fat can cause harm to our gall bladder. Fats are not soluble in water. Before dietary fat can be digested, it must be emulsified. Bile is used for this purpose. The liver continuously makes bile and stores it in the gall bladder until such time as it is needed. However, if a diet is too low in fat, that bile remains in the gall bladder. Gallstones are formed when the gallbladder is not emptied on a regular basis. In people who consume too little fat, bile is not used, and therefore, it remains unused in our gallbladder, where it stagnates. In time, sludge' collects and forms small stones which can continue to grow in size. "The speed with which this happens was dramatically demonstrated in a trial at several American University hospitals. None of the subjects had any sign of gallbladder disease at the start of the study. However, after only eight weeks of low-fat dieting, more than a quarter developed gallstones, (Groves, nd).

Fat-soluble vitamin deficiencies are another serious health risk associated with very low fat in the diet. Vitamins A, D, E, and K are fat-soluble vitamins get broken down and absorbed by fat. for example, a no-fat diet in very young children or for extended periods of time in adults can lead to a vitamin A deficiency, which is a leading cause of blindness as well as learning and memory problems. "When vitamin A lacks during gestation, as it is for most mothers in our fat-phobic society, children may be set up for abnormal behavioral patterns later in life" (Onusic, 2013).

For those whose consume lots of nutrient-rich vegetables that are high in vitamin A, D, E, and K, but remain on a no-fat diet, their deficiencies are caused by the inability to absorb the fat-soluble vitamins. Whereas vitamin A is a fat-soluble vitamin, the lack of fat prevents our body from absorbing and using it.

Extensive studies date back as far as the 1930s have confirmed the need for healthy fat in our diets and identified unhealthy fats as the cause of both confusion and many modern-day epidemics.

"During the past several decades, reduction in fat intake has been the main focus of national dietary recommendations to decrease the risk of coronary heart disease (CHD). Several lines of evidence, however, they have indicated that types of fat have a more important role in determining the risk of CHD than the total amount of fat in the diet. Metabolic studies have long established that the type of fat, but not the total amount of fat, predicts serum cholesterol levels. In addition, results from epidemiologic studies and controlled clinical trials have indicated that replacing saturated fat with unsaturated fat is more effective in lowering the risk of CHD than simply reducing total fat consumption. Moreover, prospective cohort studies and secondary prevention trials have provided strong evidence that an increased intake of n-3 fatty acids from fish or plant sources substantially lowers risk of cardiovascular mortality," (Hu, 2001).

"The mature skeleton is a metabolically active organ that undergoes continuous re-modeling by a process that replaces old bone with new bone. In healthy adults, bone resorption and formation are balanced, and a constant level of bone mass is maintained. Over the past years, the body of evidence to support the notion that dietary long-chain polyunsaturated fatty acids (LCPUFAs) with a chain length longer than 18C are beneficial for bone health has been growing. Very early research showed that a deficiency in LCPUFAs could affect bone: In 1931, Borland and Jackson reported that essential fatty acid (EFA)-deficient animals were found to develop severe osteoporosis coupled with increased renal and arterial calcification. Studies dating back to 1946 reported that individuals with osteoporosis frequently also had ectopic calcification in other tissues, particularly intervertebral discs, arteries, and kidneys. More recently, pathological fractures were reported in newborn rats following dietary EFA deficiency. In a definitive review by Kruger and Horrobin, it was suggested that PUFAs of the n-3 series, as well as the n-6 fatty acid gamma-linolenic acid (GLA), may prove beneficial when consumed in appropriate amounts. In addition, it has been shown that a reduction of the n-6/n-3 PUFA ratio could result in increased bone strength in animals and in humans (Kruger, 2010).

99

Low levels of vitamin D are associated with increased risk of depression and panic and affect portions of the brain involved in learning and memory, as well as motor control (McCann, 2007).

Vitamin D strongly influences the production of serotonin, the molecule of will power, and delayed gratification. Decreased serotonin activity can lead to an inability to create and act on well-formed plans. There are many vitamin D receptors in the brain. Bright light going through the eyes increases serotonin production, sunglasses block this effect, and sunscreen prevents the vitamin D formation in the skin. Studies show that the production of serotonin is directly related to the duration of bright sunlight. Sunbathing and exposure to bright light during the day can have a similar effect to antidepressants, (Korb, 2011)

Research has shown that vitamin K is involved in the health of our nervous tissue, and it contributes to the biological activation of proteins involved in many cellular functions such as cell growth, survival, and the aging process. Vitamin K_2 can affect psychomotor behavior and cognition. All these vitamins were consumed at very high levels in primitive diets (Price, 2008). Today, due to disastrous dietary advice, most people avoid the nutritional sources of these critical nutrients: egg yolks, butter, organ meats, meat fats, goose and chicken liver, cod liver oil, fish eggs, and oily fish, and some fermented foods like sauerkraut," (Onusic, 2013).

When consuming fats from organic sources, those foods predictably contain many other macronutrients and micronutrients that can help us use all of the nutrients effectively. Certain diseases may increase the need for healthy fats. Those with Parkinson's disease shake and burn more calories; therefore, they need additional healthy fat for energy.

The bottom line is, no nutrients should be eliminated from the diet, including fats. Health problems associated with fat intake are due to the quality of fat and not the consumption of healthy fats.

Key Points

♣ A child's diet deficient in nutrients, in addition to inconsistent eating habits, is a high risk for cognitive impairment, obesity, and other long-term problems.

♣ Our body breaks down macro- and micronutrients into tiny particles. As small particles, they are used as ingredients and building blocks to manufacture supplies needed for the body to function.

♣ Even a small imbalance in micronutrients can cause significant health problems.

♣ All nutrient deficits that affect the physiological processes of the brain can cause less efficient communication between our brain cells and other organs.

♣ Cheaply processed foods have become the gateway to many other health problems over the past decade. People fed high-volumes of poor-quality foods are more likely to become overweight with malnutrition, which leads to chronic illnesses.

♣ The number of calories needed to survive is based on the weight and activity level of each person and animal. During times of growth, repair, and healing, your body requires additional high-quality calories, especially protein, to aid in the process of healing itself.

♣ Our body needs more macronutrients than micronutrients, but both are equally important Micronutrients taken in large quantities can cause severe mental and physical health problems, including heart problems and violent behavior.

♣ Organic food sources consistently contain the same nutrients. Therefore, they are the most dependable source of nutrients.

♣ Our body needs a constant assortment of nutrients in sufficient quantities to build supplies necessary to regularly restore, update, and replace every part of our body, including skin, blood cells, bone, and cartilage.

♣ Some nutrients are *non-essential* because a healthy body will efficiently use protein, carbohydrate, fats, and micronutrients to manufacture these vital components. Therefore, we do not need to consume those specific nutrients in their complete form. Whereas, *essential* nutrients need to be eaten regularly because our body is not capable of manufacturing them.

♣ Multiple studies have proven that DNA and RNA from foods containing Genetically Modified Organisms (GMO) have transgenetic fragments that can mix with DNA during cell division and replication, causing that person or animal's DNA to mutate.

♣ Many environmental exposures, such as pesticides, genetically altered organisms, and chemicals, can damage your DNA.

♣ There is a considerable threat of mutations to your original healthy cells when your natural DNA and RNA are exposed to mutant fragments from transgenetic materials such as that found in GMO food.

♣ Genotoxic agents or processes alter the structure, information content, or segregation of DNA. Genotoxicity interferes with your routine DNA replication processes, which ultimately result in new instructions telling our body to act in a way that may help or harm your health.

♣ In addition to organic DNA and RNA in all living things, Genetically Modified Organisms(GMO) are the third type of nucleic acid that has risen to enormous proportions in the foods sold to American consumers. GMO foods and chemical additives that contain mutations do not occur naturally; they are a manufactured commodity made by food scientists and engineers.

♣ Amino acids are used to make nucleic acids, fat, energy, hormones, enzymes, neurotransmitters, and many other life-sustaining supplies.

♣ Our body is continuously building and restoring itself, whereas protein is the primary nutrient responsible for repairing and healing our body.

♣ Amino-acids/ Proteins are vital chemically-reactive building blocks. Their quality is at least as important as the number of proteins consumed. Poor quality and /or insufficient amounts of any amino acids can cause many health problems.

♣ Processed foods remove natural starches and fibers found in carbohydrates and also remove its natural fat and proteins. They replace those vital nutrients with simple carbohydrates used to restore its texture and taste. These simple carbs do not contain vitamins, minerals, or fiber. Replacing saturated fats with simple carbs increases our risk of heart disease, high LDL cholesterol, and type 2 diabetes.

♣ Carbohydrates are the sugars, starches, and fibers found in fruits, grains, vegetables, and milk products. Each kind of carbohydrate performs distinct jobs in the body.

♣ For our body to function properly and have enough energy to meet its needs, one-third of calories consumed should come from healthy organic fats.

♣ Multiple research studies indicated that types of fat have a more important role in determining the risk of CHD than the total amount of fat in the diet. Metabolic studies have long established that the type of fat, but not the total amount of fat, predicts serum cholesterol levels. In addition, results from epidemiologic studies and controlled clinical trials have indicated that replacing saturated fat with unsaturated fat is more effective in lowering the risk of CHD than simply reducing total fat consumption. Moreover, prospective cohort studies and secondary prevention trials have provided strong evidence that an increased intake of n-3 fatty acids from fish or plant sources substantially lowers the risk of cardiovascular mortality

References

110th Congress. (2008). *H.R. 992 - Cloned Meat Act.* Washington, D.C.: USGov.com.
Aminoacidstudies.org. (unk). *Cysteine.* Retrieved from aminoacidstudies.org:
    https://aminoacidstudies.org/l-cysteine/

Appel, L. S. (2005). Effects of protein, monosaturated fat, and carbohydrate intake on blood
    pressure and serum lipids. *JAMA v.294 (19)*, 2455-2464. Retrieved from JAMA v.294
    (19).

Arendt, E. Z. (2013). Amaranth. In E. Z. Arendt, *Cereal Grains for the Food and Beverage
    Industries* (pp. 439 - 473). Cambridge: Woodhead Publishing.

Barkley, W. B. (1979). *Laboratory Safety Monograph A Supplement to the NIH Guidelines for
    Recombinant DNA Research .* Bethesda, MD: U.S. DEPARTMENT OF HEALTH,
    EDUCATION, AND WELFARE Public Health Service National Institutes of Health.

Behar, J. (2016). *Not all proteins are created equal: The importance of complete quality
    protein.* Retrieved from World health network.net:
    https://www.worldhealth.net/forum/topic/3534/

Calculateme.com. (2019). *Convert ounces of butter to tablespoons.* Retrieved from
    Calculateme.com: https://www.calculateme.com/butter/ounces-of-butter/to-
    tablespoons/

Cell Biolabs Inc. (2019). *DNA damage: Cause and effect.* Retrieved from Best Rank:
    https://www.cellbiolabs.com/DNA-Damage-Causes-Effects#

Clavin, W. (2017). *https://phys.org/news/2017-02-electrons-dna-wire-replication.html.*
    Retrieved from California Institute of Technology: https://phys.org/news/2017-02-
    electrons-dna-wire-replication.html

Collingwood, J. (2018). *Brains of children with ADHD show protein deficiency.* Retrieved from
    PsychCentral: https://psychcentral.com/lib/brains-of-children-with-adhd-show-
    protein-deficiency/

Convert-to.com. (2019). *Extra virgin olive oil converter.* Retrieved from Convert-to.com:
    http://convert-to.com/549/cold-pressed-extra-virgin-olive-oil-with-nutrients-amounts-
    conversion.html

Eat This Much Inc. (2019). *Organic Whey Protein.* Retrieved from Eat This Much Inc:
    https://www.eatthismuch.com/food/nutrition/organic-whey-protein,122505/

Fang, Z. Z. (2014). Genotoxicity of Tri- and Hexavalent Chromium Compounds In Vivo and Their Modes of Action on DNA Damage In Vitro. *PLOS, a PEER review journal, 9(8)*, e103194.

FDA. (2018). *Final determination regarding partially hydrogenated oils.* Silver Springs, MD: Food and Drug Administration.

Fulgoni. (2008). *Current protein intake in America: analysis of the National Health and Nutrition Examination Survey, 2003 2004.* Retrieved from The American Journal of Clinical Nutrition, Volume 87, Issue 5, 1 May 2008, Pages 1554S 1557S: https://academic.oup.com/ajcn/article/87/5/1554S/4650421

GMO Awareness. (2014). *Does Your Body Absorb Genetically Engineered DNA?* Retrieved from GMO Awareness: https://gmo-awareness.com/2014/01/20/does-your-body-absorb-genetically-engineered-dna/

Greenwood, V. (2018). *How CRISPR is spreading through the animal kingdom.* Retrieved from Nova: https://www.pbs.org/wgbh/nova/article/crispr-animals/

Groves, B. (nd). *Dietary Causes of Gallstones Information.* Retrieved from Second.opinions.co.uk: http://www.second-opinions.co.uk/gallstones.html#.XEcacvZFyH8

Hernandez, C. (2019). *Overweight? You still have a serious fat deficiency.* Retrieved from The Healthy Home Economist: https://www.thehealthyhomeeconomist.com/fat-deficiency/

Ho, M. R. (1999). *Unregulated Hazards 'Naked' and 'Free' Nucleic Acids.* Retrieved from Science in Society: http://www.i-sis.org.uk/naked.php

Hu, F. M. (2001). Types of dietary fat and risk of coronary heart disease: a critical review. *J Am Coll Nutr.* , 5 -19.

Immunehealthscience.com. (2018). *Cysteine.* Retrieved from Immunehealthscience.com: http://www.immunehealthscience.com/cysteine.html

Infoplease. (2018). *Fats and Fatty Acids.* Retrieved from Sandbox Network: https://www.infoplease.com/science-health/guide-fats/fats-and-fatty-acids

Jackson, S. (2002). Sensing and repairing DNA double-strand breaks. *Carcinogenesis, 23 (5)*, 687-696.

Khan. A., K. S. (2017). Health complications caused by protein deficiency. *Journal of Food Science, 1(1)*, 1-2.

Killoran, E. (1992). *Good carbs vs. bad carbs. What are you eating?* Retrieved from Pritikin Longevity Center: https://www.pritikin.com/your-health/healthy-living/eating-right/603-real-food-vs-processed-whats-in-your-carbs.html

Korb, A. (2011). Prefrontal nudity. Boost your serotonin activity. *Psychology Today* , https://www.psychologytoday.com/us/blog/prefrontal-nudity/201111/boosting-your-serotonin-activity.

Kruger, M. C. (2010). *Long-chain polyunsaturated fatty acids: selected mechanisms of action.* Palmerston North, New Zealand, Pretoria, South Africa, Quebec, Canada: https://repository.up.ac.za/bitstream/handle/2263/16210/Kruger_Long(2010).PDF;seq uence=1.

McCann, J. A. (2007). Is there convincing biological or behavioral evidence linking vitamin D deficiency to brain dysfunction. *FASEB Journal; 22(4)*, 982,-1001.

NIH. (2016). *NIH guidelines for research involving recombinant or synthetic nucleic acid molecules* . National Institutes of Health, DEPARTMENT OF HEALTH AND HUMAN SERVICES. Bethesda, MD: Department of Health and Human Services; National Institute for Health. Retrieved Feb 2019, from DEPARTMENT OF HEALTH AND HUMAN SERVICES National Institutes of Health .

Norwitz, C. (2007). *Nutritional values of grains & flour.* Retrieved from Immuneweb.org: http://www.immuneweb.org/lowcarb/food/grains.html

O'Brien, E. H. (2017). *The [4Fe4S] cluster of human DNA primase functions as a redox switch using DNA charge transport.* Retrieved from Science, 355 (6327): http://science.sciencemag.org/content/355/6327/eaag1789

Onusic, S. (2013). *Violent Behavior: A solution in plain sight.* Retrieved from The Weston A. Price Foundation: https://www.westonaprice.org/health-topics/environmental-toxins/violent-behavior-a-solution-in-plain-sight/

Price, A. (2008). *Nutrition and Physical Degeneration; *8th Edition.* Le Mesa, Ca: Price-Pottenger Nutrition Foundation.

SCHS-OSHA Alliance. (2017). *Germ cell mutagenicity.* Retrieved from Alliance: An OSHA Cooperative Program: https://www.schc.org/assets/docs/ghs_info_sheets/mutagenicity%20info%20sheet_fin al_formatted%20february%202014.pdf

Sloan, F. (2007). *Lack of Serotonin leading violent, aggressive behavior.* Retrieved from Journal of Young Investigators: https://www.jyi.org/2007-november/2007/11/10/lack-of-serotonin-leading-violent-aggressive-behavior

Sparkpeople. (2013). *Calories in Organic Ground Beef.* Retrieved from Sparkspeople: https://www.sparkpeople.com/calories-in.asp?food=organic+ground+beef

Superior Fish Company. (n.d.). *Nutritional Value of Fish.* Retrieved from Superior Fish Company: http://superiorfish.com/id78.html

Szalay, J. (2017). *What are carbohydrates?* Retrieved from Live Science: https://www.livescience.com/51976-carbohydrates.html

USAID.Gov. (2016). *Whey protein concentrate commodity fact sheet.* Retrieved from USAID.Gov: https://www.usaid.gov/what-we-do/agriculture-and-food-security/food-assistance/resources/whey-protein-concentrate

USDA. (2015). *Whey protein concentrate handling.* Retrieved from USDA: https://www.ams.usda.gov/sites/default/files/media/Whey%20Protein%20Concentrate%20TR.pdf

WDF. (Unk.). *PCBs in fish and seafood.* Retrieved from Environmental Defense Fund: http://seafood.edf.org/pcbs-fish-and-shellfish

WDHS. (2018). *Polychlorinated Biphenyls (PCBs).* Retrieved from Wisconsin Department of Health Services: https://www.dhs.wisconsin.gov/chemical/pcb.htm

Weigle D, B. P. (2005). A high-protein diet induces sustained reductions in appetite, ad libitum caloric intake, and body weight despite compensatory changes in diurnal plasma leptin and ghrelin concentrations. *American Journal of Clinical Nutrition 82 (1)*, 41 - 48.

Weintraub, K. (2017). *Gene-Editing Success Brings Pig-to-Human Transplants Closer to Reality.* Retrieved from Scientific American: https://www.scientificamerican.com/article/gene-editing-success-brings-pig-to-human-transplants-closer-to-reality/

Whitbread, D. (2018). *10 Foods highest in histidine.* Retrieved from My Food Data: https://www.myfooddata.com/articles/high-histidine-foods.php

MICRONUTRIENTS

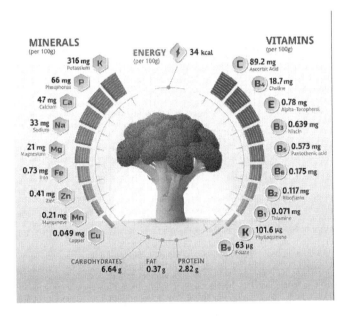

Micronutrients are kind of like seasonings and spices added to our favorite recipes. Only a small amount is needed to get their desired effect on your health. They are essential to good health and therefore, must be consumed because our body does not manufacture them. In fact, they are needed to manufacture macronutrients into useful supplies.

There are two types of micronutrients:

☺ Vitamins
☺ Minerals

Comparing vitamins to minerals, they are equally important in their own unique ways.

Vitamins

Vitamins are organic compounds found in fruits and vegetables that are essential nutrients. They must be consumed because our body does not make them, but rather uses them to manufacture internal supplies that affect health.

Vitamins must be dissolved to be used; therefore, they are either water-soluble or fat-soluble.

Water-Soluble Vitamins

Vitamins B and C are dissolved in water. They are eliminated in our urine. Neither vitamins B nor C is stored anywhere in our body. For this reason, it is essential that we consume foods containing these nutrients on a regular basis.

Water-soluble vitamins are found in fruit, vegetables, and grains. They can be destroyed by high temperatures, radiation from sunlight, and chemical exposures. For example, cooking foods, especially by boiling them, may dissolve and eliminate vitamins from those foods. Certain food additives, chemicals, and medications can inhibit your body's ability to absorb and use the vitamins derived from the foods we eat.

Water-soluble vitamins also play critical roles in our health. A deficiency of thiamine, vitamin B_1 can have serious neurological consequences. Symptoms of deficiency include depression, irritability, impulsiveness, confusion, and loss of memory. Subjects with marginal deficiencies are impulsive, highly irritable, aggressive, and sensitive to criticism. People who mostly consume foods with empty calories such as sodas, fast foods, snack foods, and alcohol are at risk for B deficiency.

A deficiency in niacin, vitamin B_3. May cause diarrhea, dermatitis, and dementia.

Vitamin B_{12} deficiency is known to cause mental disorders, including irrational anger, poor concentration, depression, severe agitation, and even hallucinations.

Up to 80% of elderly people with psychiatric diagnoses have been found to have low levels of folate. Causes of folate deficiency include chronic consumption of alcohol and/ or a large number of prescribed, over-the-counter, and illegal drugs, all of which can impair the ability to absorb folate.

Finally, regarding vitamin C, research indicates that almost any physical or mental stress significantly lowers vitamin C levels in our blood (Onusic, 2013)

The best way to keep as many of the water-soluble vitamins ingested as possible is to steam or grill foods (Justvitamins, 2014). Another way to retain water-soluble vitamins is to use water they were boiled in to make nutrient-rich soups or drinks. Also, avoid any foods or chemicals that prevent their activity.

Be aware that non-organic fruits and vegetables can be saturated with pesticides, and therefore you would not want to save the boiled water for soups and drinks. For more information about this, see the section about PLU codes and organic versus POB foods.

The benefits of water-soluble vitamins are:

☺ Vitamin B:
  o Help break protein down into amino acids
  o Converting food into energy
  o Preserving a healthy nervous system
  o Manufacturing red blood cells and DNA.
  o Aid in the development of a fetus during pregnancy; a shortage of vitamin B12 and folate can result in severe neurological damage to the developing infant.
☺ Vitamin C:
  o Immunity: Prevent and repair illnesses
  o Anti-allergic
  o Antioxidant: Protects body tissue from free radicals
  o 'Cement' for connective tissues
  o Wound healing
  o Teeth and gum health
  o Iron absorption
  o Eye health

Fat-Soluble Vitamins

Fat-Soluble vitamins are A, D, E, and K. These vitamins dissolve in healthy fats but can be inhibited by unhealthy fats such as trans-fats and chemicals that inhibit fat absorption. A diet low in quality fat can result in many fat-soluble vitamin deficiencies, whereas treatment may be simply increasing healthy fat in the diet.

Unlike water-soluble vitamins, which need to be replenished on a regular basis, fat-soluble vitamins are stored in the body fat. This means they do not need to be consumed on a daily basis because they can be stored in our body fat.

In countries where foods containing naturally healthy fats are limited, malnutrition is severe and difficult to correct. Scientists have long recognized the global epidemic of nutritionally Acquired Immune Deficiency Syndrome (AIDS) with a specific focus on Vitamin A Deficiency (VAD). VAD is the major cause of blindness in addition to debilitating loss of energy and intellect. In response to malnutrition in areas where rice is a dietary food staple, GMO scientists created rice fortified with vitamin A. They identified a gene in the DNA of Daffodils that is rich in vitamin A and injected it onto the DNA of rice. This inadvertently caused the rice to be a golden color, which gave it the name Golden Rice.

Unfortunately, the nutritional outcome of GMO Golden Rice failed to meet expectations. Vitamin A deficiency continued in areas where healthy fats were not available (Everding, 2016), (Dubock, 2014). I wonder if they had supplied healthy fat, such as olive oil or organic butter, if their vitamin A deficiencies would not have diminished.

Lack of absorbable fat-soluble vitamins has many potential deficiencies. If you experience any symptoms normally associated with these vitamins, you may want to investigate the possibility of a fat deficiency in your diet. Causes include:

☺ The quality and quantity of fats in your diet
☺ Investigate the side-effects of chemicals and food additives of frequently consumed processed foods
☺ Potential side effects of any medications you are be taking, including over the counter

Benefits of fat-soluble vitamins include:

☺ Vitamin A:
  o Aids in the growth and development of strong bones and skin
  o Promotes strong tooth enamel
  o Protect vision, especially night vision
  o Aids in the absorption of minerals
☺ Vitamin D: Is thought to be a hormone because the body produces most of it through the skin when exposed to sunlight:
  o Increases intestinal absorption of the mineral: calcium, magnesium, and phosphate
  o Promotes and protects the structure of our bones
  o Promotes immunity
  o Aids against inflammatory bowel disorders
  o Protects against depression and mood disorders
☺ Vitamin E:

- o Increases immunity and healing
- o Promotes healthy skin
- o Promotes healthy hair
- o Aids in the health of hair follicles inside ears that help to hear
- o Protects eyes
- o Acts as an antioxidant

Vitamin K1, K2, K3 (Mercola, 2004):

- o Protects the heart by preventing arterial calcification and varicose veins
- o Helps build and restore bones; prevents tooth decay and osteoporosis
- o Aids in the regulation of insulin levels
- o Helps blood clot properly
- o Aids in immunity against cancer and infectious diseases

When eating a fresh organic salad rich in fat-soluble vitamins, don't choose a fat-free salad dressing that not only lacks necessary fat to absorb those vitamins but may also be blocking their breakdown and absorption. Choose fats wisely, and you will get more vitamins and minerals from the foods you eat.

Minerals

Dietary minerals are inorganic compounds that help to keep our body and mind working properly. They are found in water, soil, and plants, but unlike vitamins, not all minerals are good for us, such as lead. Another way they differ from vitamins is that they are not destroyed by hot temperatures, chemicals, or sunlight.

Minerals are only needed in small amounts to spark essential biochemical reactions. A slight imbalance of too much or too little can cause weak muscles and bone, poor memory and mood disorders, and inability to heal. They are used to activate our enzymes, hormones, neurotransmitters, and other internally manufactured supplies.

Dietary minerals are either macro or trace (micro) minerals. They differ only in that our body needs a small amount of macro-minerals to perform their functions compared to very tiny amounts of trace minerals that are needed to stimulate their actions. Some of the better-known minerals are outlined below.

Macro-minerals

- ☺ Calcium
  - o When ionized it is an electrolyte that passes easily through cells: It activates nerve and muscle contractions and relaxation; helps form clots; Helps DNA and RNA with cell division
  - o Activates production and repair of bones and teeth
  - o Acts as a network amongst organisms: Stimulates muscle movements, nerve transmission, and vascular contraction
- ☺ Phosphorus
  - o Is part of DNA and plays a major role in the growth and overall development
  - o Helps regulate kidney functions, heart contractions, and metabolic processes
  - o Primarily stored in the bones for quick and easy access when in need of repair or restoration of our bones and teeth
  - o Aids in the conversion of food to energy
  - o Helps convert Vitamin B into energies and nutrients
  - o Help muscle contract throughout the body
- ☺ Magnesium
  - o An electrolyte needed for muscle contractions, proper heart rhythms, nerve functioning, bone-building, and strength, reducing anxiety, digestion, and keeping a stable protein-fluid balance
  - o Primarily stored in the bones, blood, and muscles
  - o Contributes to energy production in our cells
  - o Work with calcium to develop and strengthen bones
  - o Strongly affects muscle tone, endurance and pain perception
  - o Strongly supports neurological function
  - o Sodium
  - o Carry nutrients into cells and carries waste and excess fluid out of the cell
  - o Acts as a transporter of nerve impulses and contributes to muscle contraction and relaxation
  - o Regulates heartbeat regulation and blood pressure
  - o Needed to produce hydrochloric acid which is used by the stomach during digestion

- o Plays a role in regulating the body's pH balance
- o Helps muscles and nerve functions
- ☺ Potassium
  - o An electrolyte that helps muscle contractions that regulate heart rate and blood pressure, nerve signaling and delivering impulses
  - o Easily passes through cell walls to deliver nutrients and removes waste as it exits
  - o Helps regulate the body's pH level
  - o Chloride
  - o An electrolyte that moves easily through cell membranes to deliver nutrients and then removes excess waste upon exiting
  - o Helps to maintain proper kidney function by keeping fluid flowing through tissues and blood vessels
  - o Produces hydrochloric acid which activates the digestive enzyme pepsin in the stomach

Trace Minerals (micro-minerals)

- ☺ Iron:
  - o Attracts fresh oxygen into red blood cells collected in the lungs and carries to cells in our body, it exchanges the fresh oxygen for carbon dioxide, which is then used up the oxygen and returns it to the lungs to expel it
  - o Aides in the repair and replication of cells

- ☺ Copper:
  - o Helps maintain strong bones and healthy blood vessel walls
  - o Activates antioxidant reactions
  - o Helps produce energy
  - o Helps the metabolism of iron

- ☺ Iodine:
  - o Activates thyroid to produce hormones that influence our metabolic process and development of strong, healthy bones and cartilage
  - o Helps in the use of calories, thereby preventing their storage as excess fat
  - o Removes toxins from the body
  - o Aids in the absorption and use of calcium

☺ Zinc:
  o Triggers smell and taste buds
  o Helps develop and activate our immune system

☺ Cobalt:
  o Helps regulate and stimulate the production of some enzymes
  o Needed to absorb and process vitamin B12
  o Helps combat illnesses such as anemia
  o Protects and repairs the outer cover of our nerve cells
  o Helps the formation of red blood cells

☺ Fluoride:
  o Repairs and restores minerals in bones and teeth; prevents dental cavities in both kids and adults

☺ Selenium:
  o Used in antioxidant reactions that help protect the cells in our body
  o Essential for healthy thyroid function.
  o Critical to reproduction and DNA synthesis

☺ Chromium:
  o Activates enzymes that digest and store sugar and starch; boosts the effects of the hormone insulin that regulates the amount of glucose in your blood.
  o Activates digestive enzymes that metabolism of proteins and fats

Minerals and electrolytes are present in all the fluids of the body. They provide much of the spark that ignites our physiological activities into action and keeps them running. The human body is primarily made up of water and cells that need a constant supply of nutrients in order to sustain life. The combination of dietary minerals helps deliver a constant supply of nutrients to cells throughout the body while regulating our fluid levels.

It is essential that the right amount of minerals, especially those that are electrolytes, are present at all times for the proper functioning of the body systems. The slightest change in the balance of these minerals, especially the electrolytes, can cause serious health problems. Conditions such as diarrhea and vomiting can alter electrolyte levels. If the levels are significantly altered, they must be corrected quickly to avoid life-threatening consequences.

"Sometimes, an excess of a mineral can lead to mental imbalance.
An excess of copper, for example, has been implicated in Wilson's

disease, a condition with psychiatric consequences. High levels of copper can cause extreme fear, paranoia, and hallucinations. "Elevated levels of copper are found in many studies with schizophrenics, manic depressives, and epileptics. Research has established that excess levels of copper can cause violent behavior in children and youth" (Onusic, 2013).

"In research conducted over the past 20 years, we have observed abnormal trace-metal concentrations, including elevated serum copper and depressed plasma zinc, in blood samples collected from violence-prone individuals. The purpose of the study reported here was to test the validity of our observation that assaultive young males have elevated blood copper/zinc ratios when compared to a control group of young males with no history of assaultive behavior" (Walsh, 1997).

As mentioned in the first chapter, electrolytes are minerals in our blood that carry a charge that makes physiological activities occur. If there is too little or too much of certain minerals, our electricity can turn off.

Remember how the digestive system uses electricity to stimulate peristalsis? A temporary shortage in minerals can cause a temporarily shut down in our intestines resulting in an inability to process and push food through our intestines, and this can cause a blockage.

Free Radicals, Oxidative Stress & Antioxidants

Free radicals are the normal byproduct of metabolism; during the phase when nutrients are un-assembled, they have extremely high chemical reactivity to oxygen and nitrogen. Like free radicals, they are independent particles that contain unpaired electrons. Many are highly reactive and can either donate or accept an electron from other molecules and DNA. They are also derived from environmental exposures to pollution, smoke, x-rays, medications, and industrial chemicals.

The productions of more free radicals than the body can manage results in oxidative stress, which can trigger a number of human diseases (Lobo, 2010), (Bowen, unk.). Remember that our DNA can act like an electrical wire for electrons? When DNA acts as an electrical wire for the unpaired electrons of free radicals, any or all of the following can happen:

☺ It may pass directly through the cell without causing any damage.
☺ It may damage the cell, whereas the cell will repair itself.

☺ It may affect the cell's ability to reproduce itself correctly, possibly causing a mutation.

☺ It may kill the cell. The death of one cell is of no concern, but if too many cells in one organ such as the liver die at once, the organism will die.

The vitamins and minerals our body uses to counteract oxidative stress are called antioxidants. These come from our environment and the foods we consume. A balance between free radicals and antioxidants is necessary for proper physiological function.

When free radicals disrupt cell membranes, it can result in mutations that reprogram our DNA to produce diseases instead of healthy tissues. The new instructions may show up quickly or take decades to manifest itself.

The antioxidants in our body are responsible for managing the production of free radical cells and protecting our cells from oxidative stress. However, free radicals and oxidants play a dual role that generates both toxic and beneficial compounds. Therefore, the antioxidants produced in our body can also be harmful or helpful to our overall health.

One way oxidative stress develops in our body is when an imbalance between the formation and removal of free radicals occurs; when there are too many free radicals for our antioxidants to manage. This process plays a significant role in the development of chronic and degenerative illnesses such as cancer, autoimmune disorders, aging, cataract, rheumatoid arthritis, cardiovascular, and neurodegenerative diseases (Shindi, 2012) (Begley, 2012) (Pham-Hu, 2008). Oxidative stress can also cause genetic injury. This can damage the reproductive cells and be passed down to offspring, perhaps generations later. This may increase one's likeliness to get cancer, heart disease, and neurological disorders.

If a strand of DNA is damaged, the cell may repair the damage, die, or kill itself. Sometimes the cell survives but incorrectly repairs itself and then passes the genetic abnormality on to other cells during reproduction.

Key Points

♣ Micronutrients are kind of like seasonings and spices added to our favorite recipes. Only a small amount is needed to get their desired effect on your health.

♣ They are essential to good health and therefore, must be consumed because our body does not manufacture them.

♣ Micronutrients are needed to manufacture macronutrients and convert them into supplies our body uses.

♣ There are two types of micronutrients: Vitamins and Minerals.

♣ Vitamins are organic compounds found in fruits and vegetables that are essential nutrients.

♣ Dietary minerals are inorganic compounds that help to keep our body and mind working properly.

♣ Minerals are found in water, soil, and plants, but unlike vitamins, not all minerals are good for us, such as lead.

♣ Another way they differ from vitamins is that they are not destroyed by hot temperatures, chemicals, or sunlight.

♣ Minerals are only needed in small amounts to spark essential biochemical reactions. A slight imbalance of too much or too little can cause weak muscles and bone, poor memory and mood disorders, and inability to heal.

♣ Minerals are used to activate our enzymes, hormones, neurotransmitters, and other internally manufactured supplies.

References

Begley, S. (2012). *They're going to CRISPR people. What could possibly go wrong?* Retrieved from In the Lab: https://www.statnews.com/2016/06/23/crispr-humans-penn-clinical-trial/

Dubock, A. (2014). The present status of golden rice. *Journal of Huazhong Agricultural University, No. 6 (v33),* 69 - 84.

Everding, G. (2016). *Genetically modified Golden Rice falls short on lifesaving promises.* Retrieved from the Source: Science & Technology: https://source.wustl.edu/2016/06/genetically-modified-golden-rice-falls-short-lifesaving-promises/

Justvitamins. (2014). *What are water-soluble vitamins?* Retrieved from Just vitamins: https://www.justvitamins.co.uk/blog/what-are-water-soluble-vitamins/#.XHafQ_ZFyH8

Lobo, V. P. (2010). Free ra. *Pharmacogn Rev., 4(8),* 118 - 126.

Mercola, J. (2004). *10 Important facts about vitamin K that you need to know.* Retrieved from Dr. Mercola's Natural Health Newsletter: https://articles.mercola.com/sites/articles/archive/2004/03/24/vitamin-k-part-two.aspx

Onusic, S. (2013). *Violent Behavior: A solution in plain sight.* Retrieved from The Weston A. Price Foundation: https://www.westonaprice.org/health-topics/environmental-toxins/violent-behavior-a-solution-in-plain-sight/

Pham-Hu, L. H.-H. (2008). Free Radicals, Antioxidants in Disease and Health. *International Journal of Biological Science 4 (2),* 89 - 46. Retrieved from International Journal of Biological Science .

Shindi, A. G. (2012). Effect of Free Radicals & Antioxidants on Oxidative Stress: A Review. *Journal of Dental and Allied Sciences 1 (2),* 63 - 66.

Walsh, W. I. (1997). Blood Copper/Zinc ratios in assaultive young males. *Physiology & Behavior; v. 62 (2)* , 327-329.

Chapter 5

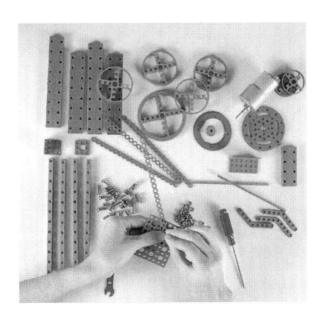

Manufactured by The Body:
Making Enzymes, Hormones, Neurotransmitters
& Much More

After you chew the food put into your mouth, and it has been dismantled, filtered, cleaned, and sorted, the tiny nutrients are packaged into each cell and loaded into your blood and lymphatic system. Nutrients are transported to and from every tissue and organ in your body.

Each organ takes only the ingredients (nutrients). It needs to make hormones that will benefit itself. Hence, high-quality foods produce high-quality nutrients that produce high-quality hormones that make each organ in our body function well. Poor quality foods produce inadequate hormones that cause organs to fail or become diseased. Diets that contain many chemicals that affect hormone production will ultimately impact the health of your organs.

Three significant chemicals that are internally made by your organs and used by your brain are:

☺ Enzymes
☺ Hormones
☺ Neuro-transmitters

Hormones travel through your blood to other cells and organs with instructions on what to do with each hormone. Neurotransmitters do the same thing as hormones but carry their instructions through the nervous system by traveling from neuron to neuron. Unlike hormones and neurotransmitters, enzymes remain inside our cells, where they act as catalysts for hormones and neurotransmitters.

Enzymes

When we eat food, our enzymes have a cyclic action. Digestive enzymes extract vitamins, nutrients, and minerals from that food. Those nutrients are used as building-blocks (ingredients) to assemble many different kinds of enzymes needed to breakdown food in the future as well as keep our blood, tissues, and organs healthy. Certain enzymes produce new cells and repair existing cells, while our metabolic enzymes deliver the vitamins, nutrients, and minerals to where they need to go. At the same time, metabolic enzymes cleanse toxins from the body. They remove old and dead material from the cells, which helps every cell in our body function more efficiently.

Digestive enzymes are produced to help us digest the foods we eat. They are secreted by the various structures of our digestive system to help breakdown food components such as proteins, carbohydrates, and fats. This breakdown into tiny particles allows the nutrients from foods to be absorbed into our bloodstreams so that they can support the functioning of all of the cells in our bodies. Digestive enzymes respond to most of our natural senses: Seeing food with our eyes, feeling it in our mouth, and smelling it with our nose. Enzymes are released in both anticipations of food and response to food. Our sensing organs can also make us lose our appetite when food is rancid, moldy, old, and many other unhealthy conditions. Merely thinking about or looking at your favorite foods is enough to get your enzyme juices flowing!

As you smell and eventually taste the food, the number of enzymes secreted increases (Bolen, 2019).

Digestive enzymes are secreted from our salivary glands, and then from the cells lining our stomach, pancreas, and large and small intestines. Different types of enzymes are secreted depending on the types of foods that we eat. They work in a cycle to breakdown and extract nutrients that help make more digestive enzymes (DeFelice, 2006):

☺ Alpha-galactosidase: Breakdown beans, legumes, seeds, roots, and soy
☺ Amylase: Breaks down carbohydrates, sugars, and starches
☺ Cellulase: Breaks down plant fiber
☺ Diastase: Breaks down vegetable starch
☺ Glucoamylase: Breaks down starch to glucose
☺ Invertase: Breaks down simple sugars
☺ Lipase: Breaks down fats found in dairy, nuts, oils, and meat
☺ Lactase: Breaks down dairy products
☺ Maltase: Breaks down complex sugars such as disaccharides to monosaccharides (malt sugars)
☺ Xylanase: Breaks down fiber
☺ Phytase: Breaks down acids to extracts minerals and helps with absorption
☺ Protease: Breaks down meats, nuts, eggs, and cheese
☺ Sucrase: breaks down complex sugars and starches

Metabolic enzymes refer to various substances within the body that carry out a variety of functions. They are a major component in the reproduction and replenishment of cells by creating energy and aid in detoxifying substances in the body. These cells are not limited to any specific region of the body. They can affect one of many bodily systems and functions. The three main jobs of metabolic enzymes are (Perfect Health, n.d.):

☺ Flush toxins from the body
☺ A catalyst for energy production
☺ Help every organ function correctly

Some of our metabolic enzymes are (Ranga, 2018):

☺ Oxidases: Changes substances to alcohols or ketones
☺ Hydrolases: Adds water to Breakdown foods and chemicals consumed
☺ Reductases: Add hydrogen to ignite a reaction

☺ Lyases: Breakdown food and chemicals without hydrolysis or oxidation
☺ Ligases: Bonds (glues) molecules together
☺ Isomerases: Convert the same molecule from one form to another
☺ Glucuronidase: Adds glucuronic acid to non-water-soluble substances which makes them water-soluble to be excreted in urine
☺ Transaminases: Add or remove amino acids
☺ Glycogen synthase: Changes glucose to glycogen in the liver. Glycogen is fuel for energy
☺ Aminoacyl tRNA synthetase: Glues together amino-acid to transcriptase RNA
☺ Lactate dehydrogenase: Changes lactate to pyruvic acid

Nuclease enzymes break apart the bonds of DNA and RNA:

☺ Neuro enzymes: Build neurotransmitters that carry messages through our nervous system
☺ Helicase unzips the double strand of DNA to allow each cell to replicate and repair itself and then transcribe that information
☺ Polymerase attaches new nucleotides to the opened strands

Ligase enzyme is another kind of enzyme that is known as a molecular glue. This type of enzyme forms a bond between the two adjacent DNA bases. Scientists use ligase in cloning to join fragments of DNA from different sources. The most commonly used for cloning is the T4 ligase, which is purified from E. coli cells infected with T4 bacteriophage (Singh, n.d.). In food preparation, it is called transglutaminase. Food glue is used to bond pieces of meat together to form one steak, roast, or another cut of meat (USDA- FSIS, 2001), (Biochem, 2002).

If the body becomes depleted of its enzymes, it becomes unable to absorb nutrients, which will interfere with its cycle of breaking down nutrients to be reassembled. When this happens, malnutrition ensues that may affect all body functions. Enzyme deficiency can be genetic or caused by medications of malnutrition.

Hormones

Hormones are chemicals produced by the cells of our endocrine glands. Hormones travel through the blood carrying instructions intended for specific target cells. Our hormones perform their unique functions by binding to particular receptors throughout our body (Home Health Network, 2019). The duties of hormones include (Nussey, 2001):
   ☺ Activate growth and development
   ☺ Repair and rebuild tissues in the body
   ☺ Regulate hunger
   ☺ Regulate reproduction, growth, and development
   ☺ Manage Mood

Some of the Hormones produced by our body are:

   ☺ Ghrelin -tells us we need more food to support our energy needs
   ☺ Leptin – tell us when we are full; when we have enough energy in storage to meet the needs of our body
   ☺ Cortisol – regulates how we respond to stress
   ☺ Melatonin – regulates sleep
   ☺ Steroid hormones – develop sexual organs, regulates fertility, and builds and restores tissues.

Neurotransmitters

Your nervous system is the record recording system. It distributes information inside and outside your body. It controls all mechanisms within your body by transmitting messages to and from your brain and spinal cord.

The nervous system is made up of nerve cells called neurons. These cells transmit signals between different parts of the body with the connection of the central nervous system, brain, and spinal cord. Neurons do not touch with each other. They use small biochemical molecules known as neurotransmitters.

Each neurotransmitter is made up of specific amino acids that must go through a series of steps that require other nutrients, called cofactors.

Neurotransmitters are the chemical messengers that broadcast signals from one neuron to the next, like a chain reaction or the phone messenger game. Target neurons receive messages through the gap between neurons.

The difference between neurons and neurotransmitters is that neurons contain messages or instructions out about the cell it resides in. Neurotransmitters are chemical messengers that help neurons to transmit their information (TheDifferenceBetween.com, 2017).

There are many types of neurotransmitters. The brain alone has 183 kinds of neurotransmitters. Neurotransmitters are made from amino acids, vitamins, and minerals. Food, food additives, and chemicals consumed greatly influence the formation and usage of our neurotransmitters (Wurtman, 1994). Timing of when we eat protein and carbohydrates throughout the day can significantly affect mood, energy, and muscle coordination and motion (Chellem, 2006).

Some of the most commonly known neurotransmitters are:

- ☺ Norepinephrine
- ☺ Epinephrine
- ☺ Dopamine
- ☺ Serotonin
- ☺ Choline
- ☺ Tryptophan
- ☺ Tyrosine
- ☺ Catecholamines

If the diet is deficient in specific nutrients, it can develop into neurotransmitter depletion (Kaslow, 2019). The depletion of neurotransmitters causes neurological and mental disorders. Many nutritional deficiencies can also be caused by medication and food additives that interfere with our body's ability the breakdown nutrients used to build neurotransmitters.

Every internally manufactured chemical is necessary for good health and the prevention of illnesses and injuries. A diet that lacks any nutrients can ignite a domino-effect of poor health.

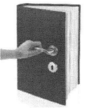

Key Points

♣ Your body uses the food you eat to make enzymes, hormones, and neurotransmitters are made by our body using the food we eat. Nutrients must be absorbed for them to perform their actions.

♣ Diets high in chemicals and processed food (food that has removed its nutrients) will cause malnutrition that results in unhealthy enzymes, hormones, neurotransmitters, cholesterol, immune cells, and other internally made compounds.

♣ Processed food and chemicals make nutrients inaccessible to your digestive system and other parts of your body.

♣ Hormones and neurotransmitters made by your body are used to send instructions to other parts of your body. Defective hormones caused by poor nutrition will send defective messages to other organs.

♣ Timing of when we eat protein and carbohydrates throughout the day can greatly affect mood, energy and muscle coordination and motion

♣ If your diet is high in chemicals and processed foods, your body may not be able to absorb nutrients when you eat nutrient-rich foods or take vitamins.

♣ A diet deficient of any nutrient can result in mental and physical illness. Processed food and chemicals can cause these nutrients deficiencies.

♣ Medications and food additives can cause a depletion in nutrients.

♣ Chemicals can reduce the absorption of nutrients, causing malnutrition.

References

Biochem, J. (2002). Transglutaminases: Nature's biological glues. *Biochemical Journal*, 377-396.

Bolen, B. (2019). *Types and functions of digestive enzymes*. Retrieved from Verywellhealth.com: https://www.verywellhealth.com/what-are-digestive-enzymes-1945036

Chellem, J. (2006). *Food mood connection*. Retrieved from Experience Life: https://experiencelife.com/article/the-food-mood-connection/

DeFelice, K. (2006). *About enzymes*. Retrieved from Karen DeFelice website: http://www.enzymestuff.com/basicswhichenzyme.htm

Gregor, M. (2015). *What is: Meat Glue,"*. Retrieved from Nutritionfacts.org: https://nutritionfacts.org/2015/04/16/what-is-meat-glue/

Home Health Network. (2019). *Hormones*. Retrieved from Endocrine Society: https://www.hormone.org/hormones-and-health/hormones

Kaslow, J. (2019). *Neurotransmitter repletion*. Retrieved from Dr.kaslow.com: http://www.drkaslow.com/html/neurotransmitter_repletion.html

Nussey, S. W. (2001). *Endocrinology*. Oxford: BIOS Scientific Publishers.

Perfect Health. (n.d.). *Enzyme Catagories*. Retrieved from Perfect Health: http://www.perfecthealthnow.com.au/bioset/what-is-bioset/enzymes-information-and-function/enzyme-information/

Ranga, N. (2018). *10 examples of enzymes with a list and their functions*. Retrieved from Study Read: https://www.studyread.com/examples-of-enzymes/

Singh, K. (n.d.). *The enzymes- tools of recombinant DNA technology*. Retrieved from Preservearticles, com: http://www.preservearticles.com/essay-for-students/the-enzymes-tools-of-recombinant-dna-technology/16170

TheDifferenceBetween.com. (2017). *Difference Between Neurons and Neurotransmitters*. Retrieved from TheDifferenceBetween.com: http://differencebetween.com/difference-between-neurons-and-vs-neurotransmitters/

Wurtman, R. (1994). Effects of Nutrients on Neurotransmitter Release. In I. o. Research, *Food Components to Enhance Performance: An Evaluation of Potential Performance-Enhancing Food Components for Operational Rations*. Washington, D.C.: National Academy Press.

Chapter 6

Nutritional Content of a Well-Balanced Diet	Function in the Body
Carbohydrates (330 g daily)	Main source of energy; fiber confers many health benefits.
Protein (100 g daily)	Major structural building blocks.
Fat (75 g daily)	Energy storage; synthesis and repair of cell parts.
Water (2000 g daily)	Solvent; lubricant; medium for transport and temperature regulation.
Vitamins (<300 mg daily)	Enable chemical reactions in the body.
Minerals (5-10 g daily)	Aid enzyme function; electrical balance; generate nerve impulses; bone structure.

How Our Body Uses the Supplies it Manufactures

Few people realize that our digestive system is the center for which all activity in our body derives its ability to function. Our body is very much like a factory, whereas every person is responsible for the quality of life he or she produces.

The materials (foods) you put into your body to make your internal supplies (enzymes, hormones, neurotransmitters, and blood cells) will be used to assemble important compounds such as cholesterol, which is needed for energy and making our immune system and hormones. These vital supplies keep your plant (body) moving and making sure you have enough of what you need.

If, by chance, you consume more supplies than what is needed, additional storage space will be needed (adipose tissue, which is known as body fat). On the other hand, if we don't consume enough materials (foods) or the materials are of inferior quality, the internal products we produce will be the low quality with poor durability.

Compare our body to a barn. Why do some last for decades and even centuries while others collapse in bad weather after only a few years? Those built with high-quality materials upon a solid foundation lasted decades. Also, their owners did not store unnecessary supplies that attract harmful pests that ultimately destroy the structure. The barns constructed initially with lesser-quality wood built upon a poorly designed foundation and then filled with supplies that will never be used will attract harmful pests that destroy the structure. These are the barns that collapse during heavy snow and rainstorms.

Our body is no different. What goes in (materials/food) is used to construct supplies and maintain our organs, bones, and other tissue. After our body breaks down the food we eat into nutrients and filters them to remove all harmful elements, each system in our body selects specific nutrients to build and restore itself. Hence, poor quality and insufficient nutrients produce poor health and an inability to maintain or restore itself. Imagine putting an addition onto your barn because you keep adding more stuff in it that will never use. Instead of using the supplies in storage, you buy more and store the leftovers. Your body does the same thing when we consume foods that have no nutritional value. We become overweight with chronic ailments that continue to store the excess as fat until we collapse.

Our digestive system is like a hardware store for all of the other systems in our body. No other system can survive without the digestive system. All other systems in our body rely on food and water. Our heart, lungs, brain, kidneys, blood, pancreas, and every other part of our body depend on the quality of the food we eat. Our diet can keep us healthy well into our old age. A nutrient-rich diet can also restore and repair our body during times of healing.

The inventory assessed by our hormones and brain determines what our current and future needs are. They evaluate the functional needs of every organ and cell in our body. In other words, our body is constantly monitoring our needs and making compounds or ingredients to meet those needs. The better the quality (nutrient levels), the lesser the quantity of food needed to extract enough nutrients. The same is true for foods with low or no nutrient value (poor bioavailability). We can consume much food that does not have the nutrients we need, and this will keep us craving more food until we consume what our body needs.

Keep in mind that calories are units of energy. You can put 20 gallons of gasoline diluted with additives into your tank to get 18 miles per gallon, or you can choose the pure gasoline that gets 25 miles per gallon. The additives may cause erosion and will only get you 2/3rds as far as the pure gasoline, which does not erode your tank. Consuming foods that are high in calories and additives, but low in nutrients will make you run out of energy faster while putting your body at risk for erosion.

Eating nutrient-rich foods and avoiding unhealthy ingredients will keep all of your systems in your body functioning at their best. A healthy diet can stop preventable illnesses before they develop.

What does all of this have to do with buying food? By understanding how the food you eat today becomes the supplies your body uses to maintain itself. As an example of how our body manufactures supplies, this next section describes how our body uses appetite regulators and cholesterol, which are only a few examples of how our body maintains itself.

Key Points

♣ The food you put into your body today will become your enzymes, hormones, and cholesterol tomorrow.

♣ Your enzymes, hormones, and cholesterol are used to build and repair every part of your body.

♣ Quality in equals quality out. When you eat a nutrient-rich diet, your body will remain healthy. If you eat foods that are high in calories and l low in nutrients, you are more likely to develop one or more preventable chronic illnesses.

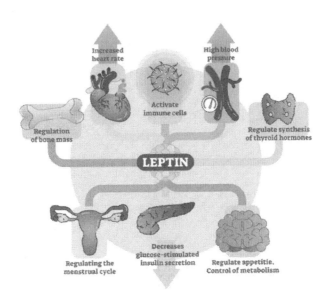

APPETITE REGULATORS

If, for a moment, you can visualize your stomach being a manufacturing plant that makes all the compounds and energy your body uses to function well. You put supplies into your stomach to be broke down, washed, and separated. When there are too few foods eaten to provide the necessary nutrients, your body will become weak and unable to sustain many functions. And, if you put too much into your stomach at one time, it will become too full to break food apart adequately. Any unprocessed food coming out of your stomach then puts a heavier workload on the rest of your digestive system and other systems that need those supplies to perform their actions. Consequently, three primary mechanisms are built into our digestive system that monitors the amount of food put into your stomach at one time and regulate appetite by continuously monitoring the amount of every supply we need. When one supply is getting depleted, hunger increases until there are enough supplies in use or storage, and then your hunger or craving is inhibited or turned off.

The first mechanisms that control hunger are stretch receptors. These are bands of muscle around the entire stomach. They warn us when our stomach is reaching its full capacity. There is a limit to how much food can fit into your stomach and be thoroughly processed. The stomach acids are released while the stomach churns its contents; together, these actions break the food into tiny nutrient particles. Stretch receptors are like rubber-bands surrounding the stomach walls. They are a proactive mechanical-mechanism that sends warning messages to your brain, telling you to stop eating when your stomach is getting too full.

You feel pain when the stretch receptors are stretched too far. This is telling you there is no more room in your stomach to fit more food, and you must stop eating until some of the food can get pushed out somehow. Aside from feeling pain when there is too much food is in the stomach, there is not enough acid to break down that much food. Like a washing machine, if the washing-machine is stuffed tightly with dirty clothing, there will not be enough soap and water to soak and wash every article of clothing thoroughly, and dirt may get caked onto all the other pieces of clothing. The churning of your stomach acts is the same way. The stomach needs moderate amounts of nutritious foods to churn adequately.

As with a manufacturing plant, if the employer increases the amount of supplies, and expects the same number of employees to disassemble and clean more of their products prior to reassembly, the quality of their product will decrease as a result of the employees being over-exerted. Stretch receptors, therefore, send warning signals to our brain to urge us to stop eating so the stomach can manage the current workload.

The other two appetite regulators are hormones. They act like instruction manuals for the rest of our digestive system, organs, and other structures. These two hormones assess (inventory) the amount of all the nutrients needed by every part of your body, and they monitor when to increase or decrease production. When more nutrients are required, Ghrelin turns on your appetite. When there is enough of every nutrient necessary to keep your body healthy, leptin inhibits your appetite. Ghrelin and leptin have a *ying-yang* effect on hunger; one balances the other. Both are released in response to instructions that come from our brain.

Ghrelin is the hunger hormone responsible for stimulating your appetite and arouses cravings for specific nutrients that your body needs at various times throughout your life. Biologically, ghrelin increases your stomach activity while decreasing your blood sugar level. When your energy level drops, your brain tells you to eat something (Cummings, 2007). It is a protective mechanism that acts like a gas gage in the dashboard of our automobiles; when your fuel gets too low, it sounds off annoying signals to warn you to fill up with gasoline as soon as possible. In your body, ghrelin signals your brain that you need nutrients and energy (Beckman, 2010). Unfortunately, it doesn't tell you specifically which nutrient is needed, but you may crave foods that have those nutrients. When a diet is missing nutrients your body needs, you may continue to feel hungry even after consuming a large quantity of food because your brain is telling you it still needs specific nutrients (English, 2002). Under healthy circumstances, ghrelin gradually increases just before meals and plays a role in how quickly we become hungry again after eating. The actions of Ghrelin (Society of Endocrinology, 2018):

- ☺ Help your brain determine how much fat your muscles need to work properly
- ☺ Signal the amygdala in the brain to feel rewarded, pleased and satisfied
- ☺ Release growth hormone to stimulate growth and rejuvenation of cells and repair your body during illnesses and injury
- ☺ Protective effects on the cardiovascular system
- ☺ Aids in control of insulin release

Getting enough sleep and not eating within a few hours of sleep also affects the release of ghrelin and leptin. Most research studies show that a balance of healthy foods can ensure we are getting all nutrients needed in the correct balance while keeping these hormones in their natural equilibrium. If one gets out of balance, most likely, the other will follow.

Leptin is the appetite-suppressing hormone made from protein by our fat-cells. These fat cells circulate in our blood and deliver messages to our brain. It is the hormone responsible for telling our brain to stop eating when there is enough energy in our blood and in storage to meet all our body's energy needs. Its primary functions are to regulate how many calories we eat, how much gets burned immediately, and how much fat will to be stored for future demands. It also controls how our energy is used (Allison, 2014). Leptin regulation of energy help (Dalamaga, 2013):

- ☺ Cognition: learning, memory, and recall, especially in children and the elderly
- ☺ Functions of your central nervous system
- ☺ Development of your immune system

☺ Regulating puberty and fertility. An undernourished, thin female will take longer to reach puberty and are more likely to have menstruation cycle problems. Reproductive growth and fat stores are vital in the regulation of reproduction (Mandal, 2018)

☺ Muscles and bone strength

Leptin sensitivity is decreased in people who are obese. As a result, satiety is not detected in spite of their high energy stores (Myers, 2010). Lower levels of leptin are detected in people with a healthy weight. Therefore, increasing leptin will not aid in weight loss.

What the hormone insulin is to type II diabetes, the hormone leptin is to obesity. People who have type II diabetes produce excessive insulin, which the body refuses to use. The same thing happens with leptin resistance. People who are obese produce excessive leptin, which their body refuses to use as an indicator to stop eating (Yadav, 2013). Instead, leptin serves to protect its levels of fat in storage.

"Leptin circulates in proportion to whole-body fat mass. In other words, a high amount of body fat results in increased leptin, which ultimately stimulates their appetite to maintain their level of fat in storage. Conversely, those with low body fat will have inhibited appetites to keep fat storage low (Freedman, 2000). Therefore, increased leptin levels do not prevent obesity (Dhillo, 2007). Research on leptin suggests that the progression of obesity is not a result of a leptin deficiency, but instead, a leptin resistance" (Bloomgarten, 2006) (Beckman, 2010).

Remarkably, there are medications to treat type II diabetes that stimulate the use of insulin already produced in our body, (Schneider, 2009), but no such remedy has been discovered and prescribed to treat Leptin resistance. This is too bad because when these three mechanisms, the stretch receptors and hormones, work as intended, we only eat as many nutrients as our body needs to sustain a long and healthy life.

Unfortunately, many food additives and chemicals, including medications and street-drugs, interfere with how these three mechanisms work. Some stimulate our production of ghrelin, causing us to eat more empty-calories than our body can use or eliminate, while others interfere with how leptin uses energy. Both cause over-eating with less energy to exercise, fight off diseases, and to manufacture adequate amounts of high-quality internal supplies necessary to remain healthy.

Remember the commercial, "Nobody can eat just one?" That may very well be true if chemicals in your food monkey with your ghrelin and leptin. Highly processed foods with additives or chemicals may trick your digestive system into bypassing your liver, your filtering system, and go directly to your pancreas, causing an overload and over-exertion. This can cascade into severe problems with the regulation of your energy and fat storage system.

Medical-providers do not routinely link obesity with malnutrition. If they did, they would be prescribing specific diet instructions to eliminate food additives known to cause those symptoms. Food additives that are GRAS are intended for healthy individuals to consume. GRAS additives are not approved outright as always safe to eat or drink because each has its own groups of people whose health could be at risk for specific symptoms when that ingredient is consumed.

Many American consumers, as patients, assume their healthcare providers would perform a thorough root-cause-analysis of their diet and environmental exposures if there were any reason to believe chemical exposures may be causing your symptoms.

If this was or is the case, then a thorough investigation of the chemicals in processed foods eaten or drank and other environmental exposures would be assessed in great detail and then mitigated (reduced or eliminated) prior to prescribing medication or surgery. Your healthcare provider would tell you what chemicals in your food are known to cause your symptoms and instruct you to avoid them while your provider monitors your symptoms to see if they go away or stay unchanged (and not increasing). Once those food and environmental chemicals are avoided, and your symptoms reduce or stop growing, then that is the treatment in itself. If your symptoms do not improve, then medication or surgery may be needed, but you should still avoid any ingredients that may cause those symptoms to come back or worsen.

Our food industry may intentionally add chemicals known that stimulate appetite for the purpose of increasing sales even when those additives are known to disrupt healthy levels of ghrelin and leptin. According to one study, "Their chemicals have few uses other than to stimulate the appetite. Big food companies are adding chemicals to already highly processed foods to increase the amount of these foods consumed, which increases sales and profit" (Hodnik, 2014).

Food additives and chemicals that undermine the development of leptin inevitably mess up insulin levels. This causes mixed messages sent to the pancreas. In its confusion, the pancreas doesn't know what to do with the excess calories, so it converts everything to fat to be stored immediately. People who continue to consume the chemicals that cause this may continue to eat too many calories that eventually deplete their leptin's ability to stop hunger. Many studies show that obese people have high levels of leptin in their system, whereas their body starts to ignore its messages; this is known as leptin resistance (Gunnars, 2017) (Myers, 2010).

Leptin resistance has three primary causes: Inflammation in the gut, inadequate fatty acids, and a hormonal imbalance. When this happens, the body can no longer process and absorb fat-soluble vitamins, and those deficiencies ignite a vicious cycle of chronic inflammation, malabsorption and vitamin deficiencies, which are the root cause of many chronic ailments that are overlooked and ignored by medical providers.

Diets low in fatty acids can be due to no-fat foods as well as medication and chemicals that impair the body's ability to use fats, which are partly responsible for feeling satisfied. Our body will continue to crave foods that have fat until it is fulfilled. In an attempt to reduce fat, many food products replace natural healthy fats with additives such as High Fructose Corn Syrup (HFCS), corn syrups and corn starches to improve the flavor, whereas studies show HFCS is directly related to leptin resistance and pancreatic tumors, (Irwin, 2010). HFCS is a simple sugar that bypasses the process of breaking complex carbohydrates down into sugar (energy). Usually, the process of breaking down complex carbohydrates helps make us feel full longer without needing to be continuously eating. The effects of fat-free foods are the opposite of what one would expect. Fat is what makes us feel satisfied when we eat, which is removed from fat-free products, and replaced with HFCS that stimulates ghrelin production, and makes us overeat, which contradicts the original purpose for eating a fat-free product.

Simple carbohydrates such as refined sugar and some sugar substitutes can cause an overload in the pancreas. They stimulate the production of too much insulin in response to the overload of sugar and causes too much energy to be removed from our blood and put into storage. The rapid drop in blood sugar quickly increases the demand for more energy, which our brain quickly releases ghrelin, telling us to eat more food to bring up our blood sugar level, and this cycle starts over. Excessive consumption of HFCS causes leptin resistance, which subsequently promotes obesity, diabetes, and pancreatic tumors (Shapiro, 2008) (Irwin, 2010).

Without much-needed healthy fats necessary to absorb fat-soluble vitamins, your leptin may become disoriented and begin to send confusing messages to the hypothalamus in the brain. If you have ever felt so stuffed that you could not fit another bite of food into your stomach, yet you still felt hungry, you probably just ate food additives that stimulated your ghrelin and confused your leptin.

When leptin resistance occurs, there are ways to restore its function. Firstly, all food additives that stimulate ghrelin and/or constrain leptin should be eliminated from the diet. Also, increase fiber intake, exercise, and improve the quality and amount of time you sleep.

Do you recall the incident in my preface when my mom told me she thought all that fat-free food I was eating was making me fat? Well, she was right! The sugars added to fat-free products stimulate appetite, and it is stored the same way fat is stored. Had I just eaten a small amount of healthy fat, like I used to do when I was thin, I would not have gained weight from all the additives put into those fat-free foods.

Oh, if only she were alive today to hear me admit she was right. Some additives trigger a craving for more food when, in fact, what we need is more nutrients.

Have you ever eaten so much food that your stomach feels ready to burst? Did you loosen your clothes to relieve the pain while you still felt hungry? If your answer is yes, it is very likely you just ate a processed food that had additives and may be genetically modified organisms, designed to stimulate your appetite. By avoiding chemicals in your diet that result in unhealthy eating habits, you can reverse many of those bad habits permanently while helping your body to repair and restore itself.

Making healthy lifestyle choices that involve your diet, exercise, and sleep can restore and repair the body.

Key Points

* Three primary mechanisms regulate appetite in humans and other animals.

* Stretch receptors are built into the lining of our stomach. They act like rubber-bands around the stomach.

* Stretch receptors are a proactive mechanism that sends warning messages to your brain. They tell you to stop eating when your stomach is full and reaching its maximum limits. It warns you to stop eating before it becomes too full to work correctly, and worse, starts to tear at the seams.

* Our two kinds of appetite hormones are regulators that act like instruction manuals for our brain: Ghrelin instructs us to turn on production, and leptin tells us to turn it off.

* When these three mechanisms, the stretch receptors and hormones, work as intended, we only eat as many nutrients as needed. Diets high in organic whole grains and high protein tend to control ghrelin better than diets high in fats.

* Remember the commercial, "Nobody can eat just one?" That may very well be true if chemicals in your food monkey with your ghrelin and leptin.

* Highly processed foods with additives or chemicals may trick your digestive system into bypassing your liver and go directly to your pancreas, causing an overload and over-exertion. This can cascade into severe problems with the regulation of your energy and fat storage system.

* Many studies show that obese people have high levels of leptin in their system, whereas their body starts to ignore its messages; this is known as leptin resistance.

* Our body will continue to crave foods that have fat until it is fulfilled. In an attempt to reduce fat, many food products replace natural healthy fats with additives such as High Fructose Corn Syrup (HFCS), corn syrups, and corn

starches to improve the flavor, whereas HFCS is directly related to leptin resistance and pancreatic tumors.

* The effects of fat-free foods are the opposite of what one would expect. Fat is what makes us feel satisfied when we eat, which is removed from fat-free products, and replaced with HFCS that stimulates ghrelin production, and makes us overeat, which contradicts the original purpose for eating a fat-free product.

* Usually, the process of breaking down complex carbohydrates helps make us feel full longer without needing to be continuously eating.

* Making healthy lifestyle choices that involve your diet, exercise, and sleep can restore and repair the body.

References

Allison, M. M. (2014). 20 years of leptin: Connecting leptin signaling to biological function. *Journal of Endocrinology*, 25 - 35. Retrieved from Journal of Endocrinology.

Beckman, L. B. (2010). Changes in gastrointestinal hormones and leptin after Roux-en-Y Gastric Bypass procedure: A review. *Journal of American Diet Association, 110(4)*, 5710584.

Bloomgarten, Z. (2006). Gut and adipocyte peptides. *Diabetes Care, 29*, 450-456.

Cummings, D. O. (2007). Gastrointestinal regulation of food intake. *Journal of Investment, 113*, 13-23.

Dalamaga, M. C. (2013). Leptin at the Intersection of Neuroendocrinology and Metabolism: Current Evidence and Therapeutic Perspectives. *Cell Metabolism 18 (1)*, 29 - 42.

Dhillo, W. (2007). Appetite regulation: An overview. *Thyroid, 17(5)*, 433-445.

English, P. G. (2002). Food fails to suppress hunger in obese individuals *Journal of Endocrinol Metabolism, 87*, 2984.

Freedman, J. (2000). Obesity in the new millennium. *Narue,404*, 632 634.

Gunnars, K. (2017). *Leptin and Leptin Resistance: Everything you need to know.*

Hodnik. (2014). *Are appetite stimulants responsible for the American obesity epidemic?* Retrieved from Iron magazine: http://www.ironmagazine.com/2014/are-appetite-stimulants-responsible-for-the-american-obesity-epidemic/

Irwin, K. (2010). *Pancreatic cancers use fructose, common in the Western diet, to fuel growth.* Retrieved from UCLA Health Sciences: http://newsroom.ucla.edu/releases/pancreatic-cancers-use-fructose-165745

Mandal, A. (2018). *What does leptin do?* Retrieved from Medical Life Science News: https://www.news-medical.net/health/What-Does-Leptin-Do.aspx

Myers, M. L. (2010). Obesity and leptin resistance: Distinguishing cause from effect. *Trends Endocrinol Metabolism, 21(11)*, 643 - 651.

Schneider, C. (2009). *Diabetes medication and care.* Retrieved from Diabetescare.net: http://www.diabetescare.net/article/title/diabetes-medications-insulin

Society of Endocrinology. (2018). *Ghrelin.* Retrieved from You and your Hormone from the Society of Endocrinology: http://www.yourhormones.info/hormones/ghrelin.aspx

Yadav, A. K. (2013). Role of leptin and adiponectin in insulin resistance. *Clinica Chimica Acta, 417*, 80 - 84.

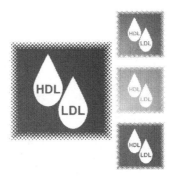

CHOLESTEROL: ~~HEALTHY OR LOUSY~~ HOUSEKEEPERS AND LABORERS

Many people think their cholesterol is partly healthy and partly lousy. As a patient advocate and health educator, I know this is erroneous and causes confusion that leads to making poor lifestyle choices with dire consequences. Therefore, everyone must understand what cholesterol is and why our body manufactures it. It is vital to life, and no animal can live without it because it acts like the fuel and oil that keeps us moving.

Everyone produces cholesterol in different amounts throughout their life. The quantity produced depends on many factors, of which some are inherited, and others are due to diet and environmental exposures.

Knowing why your body is producing too much or too little cholesterol is as important as having it treated medically because no one wants to contradict our body's efforts to maintain and repair itself. For example, cholesterol is necessary for the development of a fetus; therefore, a pregnant woman produces a lot more cholesterol during her pregnancy to support both the fetus and herself. It would not be in the best interest of the fetus or mother to take medication that reduces her cholesterol during this time because there would be enough cholesterol to meet all of the needs of the baby's and mother's health. There are many other times when cholesterol will increase to meet the needs of both males and females.

Therefore, I label cholesterol according to their functions: Housekeepers and laborers. Some act as housekeepers. These are typically called good or healthy because they keep our vessels clean and free of plaque by removing any debris in our vessels. Having enough housekeepers in our blood will prevent the risk of heart disease and strokes. The other kinds of cholesterol are laborers. These are often referred to as bad or lousy cholesterol, when in fact, they are:

- ✓ The fuel that energizes the entire body
- ✓ The cargo system that transports laborers to other organs where hormones and immune cells get made
- ✓ The ingredients that make up the structure of cell walls, help produce appetite and sexual hormones, and build resistance to diseases

Our body manufactures this waxy-like substance known as cholesterol because it is vital to our life. Some cholesterol serves as the gasoline, oil, and other fluids used to keep vehicles running. Others are like the quality of wood and hardware used to build a barn or house. Cholesterol provides the energy to every cell in our body and also helps carry out most functions. Our brain, heart, kidneys, lungs, and every other organ and tissue in our body cannot work without cholesterol. For example, if you let the gasoline-run dry in your vehicle, it stops running, and just before it stops running, all the gunk on the bottom of the tank gets into the gas lines, which can buildup in the engine (our heart) causing it to fail.

Well, the same is true with cholesterol. Therefore, none of the types of cholesterol are lousy unless you eat the most inferior quality of ingredients that are then used to make your laborers. For instance, without triglycerides and Low-Density Lipoproteins (LDL / lousy / bad), your body would wither and die. All functions would stop. Your brain would not have enough fuel to command the rest of your body. None of your organs could produce hormones needed to regulate and deliver nutrients to other parts of your body, where cholesterol is used to maintain each cell. Your body produces additional cholesterol when it detects diseases or injuries. This increase in cholesterol production is used to build your defense system. If you are unable to increase your production of cholesterol for any reason, including diet or taking medication to lower cholesterol, any disease that enters your body is free to take over. No animal can exist without cholesterol.

Imagine you own a manufacturing plant that makes gizmos. Your particular plant hires 160 employees to perform all the many tasks required to produce the gizmo's your plant makes while having enough housekeepers to maintain your building. You will need both housekeepers and laborers. If you don't have enough housekeepers to keep the plant clean, garbage will collect in the isles and workspaces, making it unsafe for the laborers and may interfere with their efficiency. Your manufacturing plant should always have at least 60 employees on hand. Having plenty of High-Density Lipoproteins (HDL), which are your housekeepers in our body, is ideal, which is explained later in this section.

Equally importantly are skilled employees who perform duties such as receiving and shipping (nutrients), dismantling parts (breaking nutrients down into macronutrients and micronutrients), clean them (in your liver and kidneys), pack and load supplies onto conveyer belt (our blood) to be deliver to other workstations (organs such as our brain, heart, kidneys and lungs) to be used however the customers desires. Our organs make hormones. Our brain uses cholesterol to energize it and perform as the command center for our entire body. Our brain is kind of like the president of our company; it commands every function in our body. It uses about 25% of all of the cholesterol in the body to perform essential tasks that keep messages to and from other organs and systems flowing well. The rest of our cholesterol is the fuel, oil, and ingredients that keep our manufacturing plant alive.

As previously stated, during normal times, your particular company needs 160 employees to keep your plant running smoothly. A competitor may only need 140 employees, or maybe they need 230 to keep their factory running smoothly. The number of employees (your total cholesterol) depends on the demands of your manufacturing plant (body). During times when the demand for gizmos goes up, more laborers/ employees (total cholesterol) will be needed to keep up with the demand.

Our liver manufactures our cholesterol. By communicating with other organs, our liver can determine how much cholesterol our entire body needs at any given time. If any part of our body becomes infected or damaged, additional cholesterol is made to manufacture immune cells. There are many times throughout our life when extra cholesterol is natural and healthy, such as during childhood and puberty. It is vital for learning and memory (retention of information) for both children and the elderly. During the times when our body needs additional cholesterol, having too low or purposely lowering your cholesterol can undermine our ability to restore and maintain our health.

Under optimal conditions, our liver used recycled cholesterol and stored fat to produce cholesterol. Less than 20% of total cholesterol comes from the food we currently eat. If a person is vegan, eats no animal products, his or her body will still produce all the cholesterol needed to sustain a healthy, well-functioning body and will increase its production when additional cholesterol is required. For this reason, the quality of fat manufactured and stored as adipose tissue (body fat) dramatically impacts the quality of cholesterol made by our liver.

Junk food laden with toxic chemicals gets converted into fat that will either be used by the liver to create cholesterol immediately or stored in our body fat until it is needed. Unhealthy fat tainted with toxic chemicals may be harmful when used to make cholesterol. When poisonous chemicals get stored in fat, their harmful effects on your body may not occur until your body uses that toxic fat, which may be years later when trying to lose weight.

Therefore, people who consume poor quality foods produce (manufacture) poor-quality cholesterol. When we eat organic, nutrient-rich foods, our liver can manufacture cholesterol in amounts that keep us healthy.

Many people confuse cholesterol with fat, which they are not synonymous. Cholesterol is either recycled or manufactured by the liver using proteins and fat; hence, its name lipoproteins. Occasionally it uses proteins, fats, and carbohydrates to make triglycerides. The amount produced depends on the body's needs for energy, immunity, and hormones. Fat, on the other hand, is consumed and broken down into fatty acids that are either used to manufacture many kinds of compounds (it is kind of like an ingredient in a recipe) or provide energy.

No animal or fish can exist without cholesterol. It is used to form cell-wall structures in every cell in our body (kind of like sheetrock and plaster). Cholesterol provides the fuel for our DNA and RNA to replicate itself. It is an essential component for vitamin D, immune cells, enzymes, and hormones to be produced. It is the Low-Density Lipoproteins (LDL) and Triglycerides that comes to our rescue when attacked by diseases such as cancer or injured with broken bones and strained muscles. These skilled laborers should not be labeled *lousy* because they are essential to fight off infections and restore our mental and physical wellbeing.

Although cholesterol-lowering medications under certain circumstances lower the risk of heart attacks or strokes, "our nation's obsession with lowering cholesterol ignores the potential psychological consequences that can occur with low cholesterol. Too low cholesterol increases the risk of depression, suicide, and violence" (Greenblatt, 2011). It also ignores the potential physical consequences of low cholesterol that may put men at higher risk for prostate cancer (Wettstein, 2017), people in general at higher risk for colon cancer (Forones, 1998), lung cancer (Zhang Y. X., 2017), and even dementia (West R1, 2008).

Our body increases its production of cholesterol during times of healing from injury or surgery. We produce additional cholesterol when fighting diseases or inflammation of our intestines and stomach (Iribarren, 1995) (Huang, 2007). More cholesterol than average is needed for those with Parkinson's disease because it helps meet the additional demands for energy caused by shaking. The development of Parkinson's disease is linked to low levels of cholesterol (Guo X., 2015) (Huang, 2007).

During puberty, cholesterol levels greatly fluctuate with hormonal changes. Cholesterol helps build strong bones and form sexual hormones. "During all stages of growth, parents should be aware of how cholesterol levels naturally fluctuate so that the interpretation of lipid levels in children are not misdiagnosed" (Bertrais, 2000).

Many women cannot get pregnant when they have too little LDL cholesterol circulating in their blood. This is because cholesterol is a primary ingredient used to build strong and healthy fertile eggs; also, it provides the energy to convert other nutrients into useful reproduce compounds needed to grow new life. During pregnancy, cholesterol levels naturally increase to meet the needs of the developing baby inside, whereas low cholesterol can cause miscarriage, brain damage, immune deficiencies, and many disabilities in the fetus. Cholesterol levels fluctuate during menstrual cycles for women of childbearing age. For this reason, cholesterol levels in women of childbearing age should always be checked at the same point in her menstrual cycle. Otherwise, her natural fluctuation that is due to her hormonal balance may be mistaken for an abnormal change in her cholesterol numbers (NIH, 2010) (Mumford, 2011).

The same is true with all animals. Healthy cholesterol improves fertility and aids in the production of healthy eggs. Keep this in mind when wondering whether chicken eggs are good or bad for you. It much depends on the health of the chicken; those raised outside where they get plenty of sunlight and eat uncontaminated real grains will produce healthy eggs. Whereas, chickens fed cow manure processed into grain for chicken feed and never see the light of day produce eggs so weak in nutrients and structural texture.

Our body and especially our brain require high-quality nutrients for itself and to instruct the rest of our body on how to manufacture the right amount of high-quality cholesterol that meets our daily needs. Everyone must maintain the right balance and understand the cause of any imbalance. The more you know about cholesterol and what your personal needs and risks are, the better you and your medical provider can determine what cholesterol levels are best for you, because too low can be as risky as too high.

Cholesterol is responsible for:
- ☺ Providing energy and structure to every cell in the body
- ☺ Protects and feeds your brain & central nervous system:
  - o The brain is the most cholesterol-rich organ in the body; it uses about 25% of your cholesterol (Orth M. B., 2012)
  - o Higher levels of total cholesterol, including the laborers, in older people, are associated with better memory and resistance to dementia (West R1, 2008)
  - o In children, "cholesterol is critical to learning and memory" (Schreurs, 2010)
- ☺ Making all of our hormones:
  - o Mineralocorticoids: Regulate sodium and potassium that are required for water and electrolyte balance
  - o Glucocorticoids: Breakdown carbohydrates; Cortisol is an anti-inflammatory hormone that helps prevent autoimmune reactions
  - o Appetite hormones: Ghrelin and Leptin
  - o Androgens (Testosterone & DHEA): Regulates libido, builds muscle mass and prevents osteoporosis, prevents memory loss and aging
  - o Estrogens: Needed for sexual development and fat storage; aids in bone and brain health, as well as thyroid function
  - o Progestogens: Regulate female fertility by managing menstruation. Also regulates body temperature; whereas, during menopause, some women experience hot flashes due to the change in this hormone
  - o Vitamin D: Helps our body use calcium and make immune cells
- ☺ Providing nutrients and energy for the production of immunity during its battles against diseases and recovering from injuries. Too little fuel can cause reduced resistance to infections and the inability to make new immune cells

☺ During pregnancy cholesterol significantly increases to support the formation of the central nervous system, developing hormones and provide energy to the fetus

☺ Aids Digestion: Creates bile salts used to emulsify fat during digestion

Healthy and Lousy cholesterol are misleading labels that interfere with American's understanding of when and why cholesterol levels naturally fluctuate throughout life, especially during times of growth, illness, and injuries. Any misconceptions about high cholesterol can lead to hasty medical decisions to lower cholesterol when our body may be producing additional cholesterol to ward-off or fight an illness or disease, including heart disease, cancer, blood infections and a host of other conditions (Casteel, 2012) (Greenblatt, 2011) (Huang, 2007) (Hu, 2001) (Iribarren, 1995) (Khanse, n.d.) (Lopez-Jimenez, 2018) (Schreurs, 2010) (Wilson R. B., 2003) (Wolfson, 2017). Or, your body may be healing strained or broken tissue inside your body. These misleading labels prevent Americans from making truly informed decisions about their health.

Perhaps the best approach and first step to securing optimal cholesterol levels are to make better lifestyle choices, especially dietary, while figuring out the cause of any imbalances.

"If the recommendation to restrict dietary cholesterol is dropped, this fits with the new way health professionals and scientists are thinking of nutrition advice. Rather than focusing on specific nutrients or compounds, like cholesterol, many nutrition researchers are focusing on dietary patterns to understand how what we eat affects health and disease risk.

Singling out the role of specific nutrients, like cholesterol, fat, protein, fiber, or vitamins, provides only one piece of the dietary puzzle. Because we eat a variety of foods and not just nutrients, all the substances in those foods interact in our body in complex ways to affect health.

Evidence is mounting that a variety of plant-focused eating patterns are cancer-fighting and promote overall health. These diets include plenty of vegetables, fruit, whole grains, legumes, and nuts, and they also lower risk for type 2 diabetes and cardiovascular disease." (AINFCR, 2015).

One six-year study of people over the age of 75 found, "high cholesterol did not predict mortality in our study population. On the contrary, low cholesterol levels were associated with higher mortality. This association seems to be only partly explained by frailty" (Tuikkala, 2010). Telling someone to lower their cholesterol without investigating the cause is like telling an over-weight person never to eat again. The dire consequences can cause worse health outcomes than the initial symptom. A better way to understand and adequately respect the types of cholesterol is to think of them as "Housekeepers and Laborers." Each type of cholesterol has very specific duties. The three primary types of cholesterol are:

☺ High-Density Lipids (HDL): Our Housekeepers keep vessels clean and free of debris

☺ Low-Density Lipids (LDL): Our laborers provide energy and help make compounds such as hormones and immune cells

☺ Triglycerides (TGC): Are also laborers that transport of HDL and LDL to cells and help make essential compounds.

Total Cholesterol (TC)

TC is the sum of all cholesterol circulating in our blood. The amount circulating in our blood is like the number of employees in our plant. We need enough healthy housekeepers and laborers to keep our manufacturing plant working well, and production sufficient to meet our customers' (organs) demand. We need high-quality workers (LDL and triglycerides) because slackers (empty calories with toxic compounds) can be a drain on any system.

The total number of all the types of cholesterol is less informative than the specific numbers because so much depends on the quality of the laboring cholesterol and the number of housekeepers available to keep our blood clean and free of plaque buildup. For instance, just having 160 employees does not guarantee high productivity. Say you hire 140 laborers to work on the assembly line, can you safely rely on only 20 housekeepers to keep up with cleaning all the work surfaces while removing trash and mopping the floors? It is better to have at least 60 housekeepers at all times and while the number of laborers can fluctuate with the demands for their labor. Therefore, making better lifestyle choices (maintaining the right balance of employees) will keep our total cholesterol at a level that meets your unique needs.

HOW TO ASSESS YOUR TOTAL CHOLESTEROL

Total Cholesterol is the sum of our High-Density Lipoprotein HDL) plus Low-Density Lipoprotein (LDL) plus [Triglycerides (TGC) that have been divided by 5].

TC = HDL + LDL + [TGC ÷ 5]; for example, HDL of 70 mg/dl + LDL 130 mg/dl + TGC [150 ÷ 5 = 30 mg/dl]= 230. Each of these individual numbers are healthy levels and yet by modern standards, TC of 230 falls into the high risk for stroke and heart disease.

Today, the American Heart Association recommendations are:
Less than 200 mg/dl = ideal
201 -239 mg/dl = borderline risk for stroke and heart disease
Greater than 240 = high risk for stroke and heart disease

Currently, there are no parameters for too low cholesterol. Many medical professionals advise 'the lower, the better.' But, too little can be as risky as too high in individuals people due to the broad array of lifestyles that may expose them to unhealthy environmental conditions (Bertrais, 2000) (Casteel, 2012) (Greenblatt, 2011) (Huang, 2007) (Khanse, n.d.) (Wilson R. B., 2003). Researchers have found that lowering cholesterol to unsafe low levels may be rare but can cause irreparable injury to muscles and kidneys (Lopez-Jimemez, 2019) (Drugs.com, 2018). In some cases, it may cause type II diabetes (Lotta, 2016).

Studies show that low cholesterol during illness can thwart recovery. "Normally, the blood-cholesterol levels outweigh the digestive system needs of the adrenal gland. However, critically ill patients may have extremely low cholesterol levels. A U-shaped curve between cholesterol level and mortality was shown" (Gui D, 1996) (Van der Voort, 2003).

"Hypolipidemia (too low cholesterol levels) is a decrease in plasma lipoprotein (cholesterol) caused by primary (genetic) or secondary (acquired by cholesterol-reducing medication) factors. It is usually asymptomatic (no symptoms) and diagnosed incidentally on routine lipid screening. The first report of hypocholesterolemia (too low cholesterol) in the medical literature was in 1911 by Chauffard and coworkers, in patients with active tuberculosis, (Wilson, 2003). Hypolipidemia is a common disorder affecting about 2–3% of apparently healthy individuals and up to 6% of hospitalized patients. It might be a marker for an underlying, serious problem. Unexplained hypolipidemia should always be investigated for a possible cause. Several clinical conditions, as well as lipid-lowering drugs, may result in clinically significant hypolipidemia. The evidence regarding the carcinogenicity of hypocholesterolemia from clinical studies in humans is inconclusive. The available data suggest that low cholesterol levels may serve as a prognostic indicator in cancer patients. Low cholesterol is a possible risk factor for ICH. Hypocholesterolemia is also a predisposing factor for infection in certain conditions as well as a prognostic indicator during sepsis. There is a positive relationship between low total serum cholesterol levels and increased mortality from all causes, particularly in critically ill patients. Hypolipidemia may predispose the critically ill patient to sepsis and adrenal failure and may carry a significantly increased risk of mortality. Currently, as we focus on aggressive management of hyperlipidemia, we should at least keep an eye on the possible complications of drug-induced hypolipidemia" (Elmehdawi, 2008).

In other words, when cholesterol levels are very low, it may be the first symptom warning that a person is fighting something off or struggling to survive.

Two very informative parameters indicating the health of your cholesterol levels are the:

✓ Total Cholesterol (TC) compared with how much High-Density Lipoproteins (HDL), which is your TC/HDL ratio.

✓ Triglycerides (TGC) compared to the amount of HDL in our blood. Like hiring employees for your manufacturing plant, having the optimal number of 160 employees, as previously indicated, is not sufficient enough to make your plant run efficiently. You must hire the right amount of housekeepers and laborers. Too few skilled laborers will have dire consequences, such as the inability to build enough immune cells and not enough to support individual cell walls.

The TC to HDL ratio is calculated by TC ÷ HDL = TC/HDL. $160 \div 80 = 2.0$. This formula tells us how much of our TC is HDL:

> ➤ 3.5 or less is healthy: There are enough housekeepers to keep our vessels clean even during times of an increase in LDL and TGC.
> ➤ 3.6 – 4.5 is borderline risky; during times of higher demand there may not be enough HDL to prevent a heart attack or stroke
> ➤ Greater than 4.5 is a risk for clogged vessels (atherosclerosis)

For example:

TC 240 ÷ HDL 80 = TC/HDL 3.1 which falls into the protective range

TC 140 ÷ HDL 30 = 4.66 falls into the high-risk range.

TCG to HDL is calculated by TCG ÷ HDL = TC/HDL. This calculation of cholesterol helps identify risks for metabolic syndrome, which is the combination of heart disease with type 2 diabetes (Cordaro, 2009):

≤ 2.75 in men
≤ 1.65 in women is ideal

For example:

o TGC of 150 with HDL of 60 in a man = 2.5 which is normal
o TGC of 100 with HDL of 60 in a female = 1.62 which is normal

Before 1994, Total Cholesterol (TC) less than 160 was considered a risk for contracting various diseases and poor healing. Normal was 160 to 260. When levels fell below or exceeded these numbers, further investigation was performed to identify the cause.

According to Dr. J. Wolfson, a cardiologist, total cholesterol has very little to do with living and dying. "Studies confirm that between 160 and 260, there is very little difference in mortality. The goal should be to find the ideal cholesterol level for each patient as an individual because the perfect cholesterol for one person is different than what is perfect for another.

Take, for instance, puberty, whereas cholesterol is essential for the construction and balance of hormones. "Lipid levels change markedly by pubertal stage, and patterns differ by sex and race. Chronological age ranges widely within a given pubertal stage and is an indicator of pubertal and the related changes in lipid levels. Pubertal development should be considered when determining screening criteria to identify youths with adverse blood lipid levels (Eissa, 2016). For women, menopause is another stage in life where lipid levels change and vary greatly by age and weight that needs to be considered when determining screening criteria" (Derby, 2009). Treating cholesterol during a time when the body is naturally increasing, and decreasing hormone levels may be undoing the body's natural defenses.

By understanding the essential functions of cholesterol, we begin to understand what effects cholesterol levels. There is a balance that either protects or harms us. There are times when higher cholesterol is desirable (Wolfson, 2017) (Lemole, 2017):

- People undergoing radiation and chemotherapy fare better
- Lower incidence of breast, uterine, prostate, pancreatic and other cancers
- Lower rate of Parkinson's disease
- Lower prevalence of neurological disorders
- In the elderly, a lower incidence of dementia

A higher cholesterol level may be a warning that something else is going on in our body. Reducing our cholesterol without knowing the cause may be undermining our body's ability to protect itself.

As an occupational health nurse, I promoted TC levels below 200 for every employee without consideration for individuality. I remember my employer rewarding employees who achieved and maintained cholesterol of less than 200. With what I now understand about cholesterol and its role in fighting diseases, employees exposed to cancer-causing agents, those working in extreme environmental conditions and those who performed repetitive activities whose TC were as much as 250 and appeared active and healthy were likely at those levels because their bodies had additional cholesterol-fighting needs that kept them that way. Advising and rewarding them for lowering their cholesterol could very well have caused harm to their health.

Rewarding employees for taking medications to lower their cholesterol without understanding why it was high, could have also undermined the employer by causing more workers compensation claims. If employees with elevated total cholesterol and high HDL were due to work exposures such as toxic chemicals or physically demanding work, lowering their cholesterol could have wiped out their immunity-defenses (Wolfson, 2017). A better service to those employees would have been:

153

☺ Education about lifestyle choices

☺ Reward employees based on TC/HDL ration and TCG/HDL ration

☺ Provide nutritious food during breaks

☺ Perform root cause analysis: Identify jobs that had more employees with high cholesterol and figure out how to reduce their exposure to those risks

TC levels that are too high or too low are telling us something about our health. When any health symptoms occur, evaluating the health of your cholesterol level is a good start to figuring out what is wrong with you. Monitoring cholesterol levels during lifestyle changes is an excellent way to see how your cholesterol reacts. This can help you and your medical providers determine whether you are at risk for heart attack or stroke versus healthy changes used to fight off a disease successfully.

High-Density Lipoproteins (HDL) – Housekeepers

HDL circulates in the blood vessels where it attracts and consumes unused, damaged, or old LDL. HDL cleans the walls of our vessels. It then uses the lymphatic system and our blood to return to the liver to recycle or dispose of the cholesterol collected. The longer unused LDL sits in our vessels, the higher the risk for inflammation and blockages, (Lemole, 2017). Therefore, increasing HDL and the lymphatic flow can improve the removal of unwanted cholesterol, thus decreasing vessel blockages and inflammation. Our HDL (housekeepers) keep the isles and workspaces clear of garbage. They bring it back to their central station where some of the garbage can be reused, and some must be thrown away because it is too worn out. If there are too few housekeepers, rubbish can build up in the workstations making the housecleaners scrub harder to get the area clean. During normal production, these housecleaners will complain they are breaking their backs to get the dirt (plaque buildup) off the workstations. But when there is an increase in production, these housekeepers cannot take on any more work, and this is when the workstations (our blood vessels) become unsafe (a risk for heart attack or stroke). Therefore, HDL (Housekeepers) blood levels are:
- Less than 40 mg/dl diminishes the body's ability to remove plaque-building lipids from vessel walls. Low levels may indicate depletion from disease activity; therefore, if HDL was previously healthy, it is

advisable to investigate why it dropped. If always low, examine life-style choices.

- 40 – 59 mg/dl is enough to maintain clean vessels while the body is relatively healthy.

- 60 – 89 mg/dl is optimal to prevent inflammation, heart disease, and strokes by keeping vessels clean.

- Greater than 90 mg/dl may indicate an autoimmune disorder in which the body produces too much as a response to erroneous information. If no disease process, then this should not be a concern.

When HDL returns to the liver, it's full of debris and cholesterol particles to be dismantled, sorted, and filtered. They are then recycled and reassembled or eliminated from the body. The particles that are too old and worn-out are sent to the large intestines to be mixed with other waste products. The recycled cholesterol particles make up 80% of our cholesterol under optimal conditions. Only about 20% of our total cholesterol comes from our current diet. The newly recycled cholesterols are sent back to cells to be used again, whereas some get transformed into bile salts that are needed to breakdown fat.

A low level of HDL in our blood indicates there are too few housekeepers in your body. They may not be able to keep up with the workload, mainly when during times when our body is repairing itself or needs additional energy. Typically, the liver creates more LDL to fight off the disease and more TGC to transport it. If there are too few HDL to clean up worn-out, old, and defective cholesterols, debris will collect in vessels and clog up cells.

HDL is made from fats and proteins that are consumed. The quality of what we consume will eventually become the ingredients our liver uses to make our cholesterol. Poor quality, stored body-fat that contained toxic chemicals when first destroyed, will get used to making cholesterol that is unhealthy.

Other factors that affect production are exercise, environmental exposures, and the quality of our sleep.

Low-Density Lipoproteins (LDL)- The laborers

LDL provides energy and structure to every cell in the body. They stimulate growth and repair in addition to providing fuel to every cell in our

155

body. Animal life cannot exist without it, whereas plants do not have cholesterol. Plants have a different internal chemical called sterols.

Not all LDL are alike. Our liver uses proteins, fats, and minerals to make LDL. Different amounts are used for various needs resulting in varying levels of density ranging from Low-Density Lipids (LDL) to Very-Low Density Lipids (V-LDL). Lipoproteins carry cholesterol and triglycerides through your bloodstream. Triglycerides are a type of very-low-density protein that's used to store extra energy in your cells. The main difference between VLDL and LDL is the percentages of the protein versus fat (Sullivan, 2019). VLDL contains more fat in addition to some carbohydrates, which makes triglycerides, whereas LDL contains only protein with less fat. While your body needs both cholesterol and triglycerides to function, having too much of either can cause them to build up in your arteries, which can increase your risk for heart disease and stroke.

LDL levels:

- Less than 89 mg/dl is too low (Cox, n.d.)
- 90 – 130 mg/dl is healthy
- Greater than 130 mg/dl is unhealthy, especially when there are too few High-Density Lipoproteins (HDL / housekeepers).

The central nervous system and brain use the majority of LDL. LDL cholesterol helps nerves communicate with each other and the brain. Defects in the production of cholesterol can lead to inadequate amounts available for healthy brain and nervous system functions. Low LDL can cause or be the warning of (Khanse, n.d.) (Orth, 2012), (Fazio, 2013), (Lopez-Jimenez, 2018), (Casteel, 2012), (Rosenberg, 2013):

- Problems with the nervous system and brain functions
  o Dementia, specifically Alzheimer's disease
  o Parkinson's disease: Research "found elderly people with LDL levels of less than 114 mg/dl had a 3.5 times higher incidence of Parkinson's than study participants whose LDL was more than 138" (Weil, 2007).
  o Huntington's disease and other neurological disorders
  o Learning disabilities in children
- Bleeding in the brain, especially in elderly people
- Depression, anxiety and mood disorders
- Infertility, low birth weight, and premature births

- Hormone imbalance: Hyperthyroid activity
- Degenerative disease of the retina in the eyes
- Vitamin A, D, E and K deficiencies
- Immune deficiency and reduced ability to fight off infections:
    o There are significantly fewer circulating white blood cells in people with low cholesterol. Patients with low LDL have fifteen times higher risk of developing cancer
    o Individuals with LDL cholesterol less than 70 mg/dL are five times more likely to develop sepsis
    o The lower the levels of LDL, the higher the risk for respiratory tract infections, especially elderly males. Low LDL increases the risk to all types of infections

High LDL used to be thought to prevent cancer. Many scientists today are revisiting the concept that a high LDL may indicate exposure to a disease that is being fought off or in someone who has early stages of a disease, their body has been fighting it for a while. When normal LDL levels rise, the liver produces more LDL and TGC to meet the increased demands of the body, (Pekkanen J1, 1994), (Casteel, 2012).

One example of how a chain of events can lead to high cholesterol is people who smoke cigarettes, marijuana, and other products high in cancer-causing chemicals.

You may cynically ask, how can smoking cause high cholesterol? Well, it inadvertently does so. The body uses cholesterol to manufacture its immune system and fight off diseases. When someone smokes cigarettes, they are exposing their lungs to a cancer-causing agent. Everyone's lungs are a potential portal of entry for illnesses and allergens because this is where carbon dioxide gets exchanged with new oxygen that may contain chemicals. Blood carries this newly oxygenated blood with its cancer-causing chemicals to other organs in our body. When someone's body detects infections, their liver produces more LDL to prevent and fight off cancer tumors. The increased production of cholesterol is a protective mechanism, whereas increased LDL and TGC levels during this time are beneficial to the body.

The type of LDL produced can make the difference of whether this high LDL saves or harms that smoker.

If the smoker is very active with a few other environmental exposures and consumes a diet high in healthy proteins and fats, their high levels of cholesterol will protect him or her from developing cancer. Most likely, these smokers have a TC/HDL that is less than 3.5.

But if the smoker has one or more factors that cause the liver to produce more V-LDL, that increase may clog arteries resulting in heart disease while the body is fighting cancer. Lowering cholesterol during that time may prevent heart disease while it is also preventing the body from raising enough immunity to fight cancer. Factors that may impair the quality of LDL include:

- Exposed to other cancer-causing agents:
  o In the environmental
  o Food additives and chemicals
- Poor diet: Too little or poor-quality protein and fat

In other words, smokers who have poor eating habits and sedentary lifestyles are likely to experience heart and strokes when exposed to infectious diseases, because there are too few HDL to keep their vessels clean, whereas those who eat healthily and are active may never get sick even though they smoke (Pekkanen J1, 1994).

Multiple problems can cause low LDL:

- Heredity of genes that prevent the formation of LDL
- Iatrogenic: Prescribed medication to lower cholesterol such as statins
- Liver disease interfering with cholesterol production
- Infection and injuries that use up our immune system
- A mediocre diet can cause malnutrition.
  o Poor-quality food that comes from over-processed grains, plants, and animal products
  o Added chemicals that prevent or bypass the production of cholesterol
  o Diets low in good-fats or ones that eliminate all fats can lead to fat-soluble vitamin deficiencies. Fat is necessary for fat-soluble vitamins to be absorbed.
  o An example of how additives can cause malnutrition is: Eating a salad rich in vitamin A with a fat-free salad dressing can reduce the number of nutrients absorbed from that salad. A healthy option is olive oil and vinegar to facilitate the use of that fat-soluble vitamin A.

TRIGLYCERIDE CHOLESTEROL (TGC)

Triglycerides are a type of blood-fat or lipid. They make up most of your body's fat deposits, as well as what accumulates around your waist. Our liver and pancreas play important roles in metabolizing triglycerides. Gut health is also important because our microbiota helps control levels of Triglycerides (TGC) and High-Density Lipoproteins (HDL).

TGC is a type of fatty acid used to transport and store energy. TGCs are released into our blood, where they bind with HDL and LDL to transport life-sustaining energy and transmit messages to target cells, organs, and tissues throughout our body. It then helps carry HDL back to the liver. In this respect, TGC's in healthy numbers are important to our health.

TGC/HDL ratio (TGC ÷ HDL) is a powerful tool to estimate your risk for metabolic syndrome, which is a cluster of risk factors for insulin resistance, type 2 diabetes, and cardiovascular disease. A large study performed in Spain found TGC/HDL ratio values >2.75 in men and >1.65 in women to be a strong predictor for metabolic syndrome diagnosis. TG/HDL ratio was also found to have a high predictive value of a first coronary event regardless of the Body Mass Index (BMI). These risk factors include" (Cordaro, 2009):

- ☹ High blood pressure
- ☹ High triglycerides (TGC) with low level (below 60 mg/dl) high-density lipoproteins (HDL/housekeepers)
- ☹ Problems with high or low glucose levels
- ☹ Fat collected disproportionately around the waist compared to the rest of the body; whereas fat equally distributed all over the body is not a risk factor

A fasting blood test (whereas you have not eaten anything for at least 12 hours before the test) is the best way to get the most accurate assessment of your triglycerides. Other criteria that influence TGC levels should be part of a root-cause-analysis investigated before treating high cholesterol levels. By doing so, you can identify and treat the cause instead of just the symptom. Any other way to look at this is if the front passenger tire of your car goes flat for the third time this month, would you want to patch it again (treat the symptom) or get a new tire (fix the problem)?

Medical tests that may help with an accurate diagnosed for high cholesterol include (Williams, 2017):

- ☺ Thyroid hormones: Even borderline low thyroid hormone function is associated with high triglycerides and metabolic syndrome.
- ☺ Test testosterone levels: Low testosterone levels and metabolic syndrome go together.

☺ Compare cortisol levels and HDL levels. High cortisol levels with low HDL levels in critically-ill patients in multi-system failure had adrenal insufficiency causing their inability to overcome their illness, (Van der Voort, 2003), (Bochem, 2013).

☺ Liver and kidney function studies and pancreatic enzyme (lipase and amylase) levels; when our liver, kidneys, or pancreas are compromised, we may have trouble metabolizing lipids and triglycerides.

☺ Rule out any potential diseases that your body may be fighting off.

☺ Make sure you have not eaten in the last 12 hours.

☺ Pregnancy test: All cholesterol increases to support both the baby and mom

☺ For women of childbearing age, cholesterol should always be checked at the same point in the menstrual cycle, so fluctuations due to hormonal changes are not mistaken for other causes

When calculating TGC into the total cholesterol (TC) formula, TGC is divided by five, $[150 \div 5 = 30]$. Levels are:

- No levels are considered too low by most medical providers
- Normal: Less than 150 milligrams per deciliter (mg/dL) or less than 30.
- Borderline high: 150 to 199 mg/dL or 30 to 40
- High: 200 to 499 mg/dL or 40 to 100
- Very high: 500 mg/dL or above 100

Unlike HDL and LDL, TGC's come from both animals and plants. The liver converts fats and carbohydrates into useful forms of fat that our blood can use instantly for energy. Some of this fat gets saved and stored in fat cells to be used as needed. In between meals, hormones, such as cortisol, release TGC to maintain a constant supply of energy all day long without the need to eat continuously. Excess calories and low levels of exercise are the primary causes of chronic high triglycerides.

Many high-processed foods don't need to be digested or filtered by the liver. When consumed, they go directly to the pancreas. When the pancreas is overwhelmed with too much sugar and starch, it converts it to fat and puts it into storage (body fat). The buildup of excess fat and triglycerides can lead to obesity, diabetes, and organ failure (liver, pancreatic, kidney, and heart disease). Most of the fats in American foods, including trans-fats, margarine, and oils, are in triglyceride form. Excess calories, alcohol, and sugar in the body turn into triglycerides and stored in fat cells throughout the body.

Blood triglyceride levels are typically high after you eat. Therefore, you should wait twelve hours after eating or drinking before you have your triglyceride levels tested. Many other factors affect blood triglyceride levels, including alcohol, diet, menstrual cycle, time of day, and recent exercise. When checking cholesterol levels, be aware these factors can affect the accuracy of your cholesterol levels. If triglyceride levels are chronically high or low, it is a good idea to look for causes. Do you always fast twelve hours before being tested? If you are a female, do you check cholesterol levels at the same time during the menstrual cycle? Do you consume excessive calories or high processed foods during the days before testing? Causes of too low TGC levels include:

- Malnutrition: Not enough nutrients to keep the body healthy
- Diets too low in healthy fats
- Hyperthyroidism
- Malabsorption: Nutrients are not absorbed and therefore not used
- Medications
- Food additives, low-fat foods, and ingredients that block fat absorption

TGC levels below 50 mg/dl [TGC 50 ÷ 30 = 1.4] are a serious risk for, (Andre, 2017), (Perkins, 2017):

- Deficiencies in fat-soluble vitamins A, D, E, and K
- Heart disease
- Stroke
- Insulin resistant diabetes
- Leptin resistance
- Poor clotting
- Hormone imbalances

Ways to Lower Triglycerides (Williams, 2017):
- Change your diet:
  - A plant-based diet low in refined carbohydrates (see the section on carbohydrates)
  - Avoid refined sugar and fruit juices
  - Eat more wild-fish
- Add healthy fats and oils: Avocados, olives, hazelnuts, almonds

- Cut back on alcohol. Drinking promotes liver metabolism of VLDL, which is the primary source of triglycerides
- Lower carbohydrates. If you're prone to insulin resistance, excess carbs can metabolize into triglycerides. Eliminate refined sugar and fruit juices because they quickly turn into triglycerides
- Exercise regularly. Ramping up your activity raises HDL and lowers triglycerides. Taking a walk after dinner may help prevent triglycerides from spiking
- Eat foods rich in niacin, which can boost HDL by as much as about 30% while lowering triglycerides. Some foods rich in niacin in just a serving of 3 to 8 ounces a day are chicken, liver, tuna, turkey, salmon, sardines, organic grass-fed beef, sunflower seeds, peanuts, green peas, brown rice, mushrooms, avocado, sweet potatoes, and asparagus (Link, 2018).

OPTIMIZING CHOLESTEROL MANAGEMENT

Cholesterol needs vary significantly between people. Healthy fats are essential for the learning and development of the mind and body of children. As we age, healthy cholesterol protects memory and prevents dementia (Schreurs, 2010). And throughout our life, cholesterol provides energy, immunity, and hormones that keep us active and happy.

Environmental exposures, organic and industrial foods, and lifestyle choices all play significant roles in our body's use of cholesterol. What is high or low levels of cholesterol in one person may be normal or advantageous for another; therefore, it is important to know what your baseline cholesterol is to compare future levels with those numbers. If your cholesterol numbers change, it is easier to investigate the cause when you know what your usual cholesterol numbers were and when was the last time your cholesterol was at that level.

Our body is constantly monitoring and restoring itself. Therefore, it is wise for everyone to know as much about how their body uses the foods it consumes. What is Generally Recognized As Safe (GRAS) is *NOT* always be safe for everyone! By blindly trusting the FDA without understanding your body is a risky approach to staying healthy.

Lifestyle choices are a crucial part of maintaining optimal cholesterol levels. These include (Lemole, 2017):

☺ Diet:
  o Eat plenty of vegetables
  o Eat more fish
  o Add healthy fats and oils
  o Consume organic fat products in moderation
  o Avoid fat-free foods and imitation fats that substitute chemicals for healthy fats
  o Lower carbohydrates and avoid sugar and fruit juices. If you're prone to insulin resistance, excess carbs can metabolize into triglycerides. Eliminate refined sugar and fruit juices because they quickly turn into triglycerides
  o Eat foods rich in niacin, which can boost HDL by as much as about 30% while lowering triglycerides. Some foods rich in niacin in just a serving of 3 to 8 ounces a day are Chicken, liver, tuna, turkey, salmon, sardines, organic grass-fed beef, sunflower seeds, peanuts. green peas, brown rice, mushrooms, avocado, sweet potatoes, and asparagus, (Link, 2018)
  o Eat foods that promote HDL formation: Olive oil, avocados, beans, nuts and legumes, whole high-fiber organic grains, vegetables and fruits, flax seeds, and red wine in moderation
☺ Cut back on alcohol. Drinking promotes liver metabolism of very-low-density lipoproteins (VLDL), which is the primary source of unhealthy triglycerides
☺ Exercise regularly. Ramping up your activity raises HDL and lowers triglycerides. Taking a walk after meals may help prevent triglycerides from spiking. An estimate of how much exercise is:
  o Less than 5000 steps daily are sedentary, which is a risk for illness
  o 5000 to 10,000 is moderately inactive
  o 10,000 to 15,000 is enough to maintain optimal health
  o Greater than 15,000 increases lymph drainage, increased HDL, prevents diseases and improves bone and muscle strength
☺ Increasing lymphatic flow can prevent or reduce atherosclerotic plaques and promote healthy cholesterol levels. Ways to increase flow are:
  o Exercise can triple the flow
  o Yoga

- o Drinking water: Divide your weight in half, and that is the daily recommended number of ounces of water we should consume daily
- ☺ Stress modification can decrease cortisol and epinephrine levels, which can improve our mood, which ultimately helps us make better choices about everything in our lives.
- ☺ Sound quality sleep:
  - o At least six hours a night improves retention and recall of daily activities
  - o Children who get 8 -10 hours of quality sleep learn, retain, and recall information better
  - o Healing occurs during sleep; therefore, additional sleep is needed when recovering from illnesses.
- ☺ Work with your healthcare professionals to help make informed decisions that improve your health:
  - o If cholesterol levels are high or low, investigate the cause and what specific numbers indicate.
  - o Find out what environmental exposures are common in your community and what you can do to reduce your risks
  - o Identify dietary habits that may harm your health and discuss ways to eliminate them
  - o If prescribed medication, ask your provider:
    - What do you need to reduce your need for that medication? What must you do to have the doctor stop that medication?
    - What type of LDL do you have?
    - Do you have any active disease processes that may be causing you increased LDL? If so, will lowering your cholesterol by taking medication, undermine your body's ability to fight that disease?
    - What food additives and chemicals can cause cholesterol to be too high or too low?

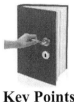

Key Points

* ♣ Misconceptions about cholesterol can lead to making poor lifestyle choices

* ♣ No animal or fish can survive without Cholesterol. It is essential to maintain optimal health.

* ♣ A good way to remember the types of cholesterol is: Housekeepers are HDL that keep our vessels clean; Laborers are LDL and triglycerides that: Provide energy to the entire body, make hormones, and helps to build our immune system.

* ♣ Our body uses high-quality foods to manufacture the right amount of high-quality cholesterol. Poor quality food and result in poor quality cholesterol in unhealthy numbers that are out of balance with each other.

* ♣ Everyone needs to maintain the right balance and understand the cause of any imbalance. The more you know about cholesterol, what your personal needs and risks entail, the better you and your medical provider can determine what cholesterol levels are best for you, because too low can be as risky as too high.

* ♣ High total cholesterol may be the first indication that the body is fighting off a disease, repairing itself, or merely needing additional energy from overexertion.

* ♣ When toxic chemicals are stored in fat, their harmful effects on your body may not occur until your body uses that toxic fat, which may be years later when trying to lose weight.

* ♣ Low-Density Lipoproteins (LDL) and Triglycerides come to our rescue when your body is attacked by diseases such as cancer or injured with broken bones and strained muscles. These skilled laborers should never be thought of as *lousy* because they are

necessary to fight off diseases and restore our mental and physical wellbeing.

♣ Cholesterol levels fluctuate during menstrual cycles for women of childbearing age. For this reason, cholesterol levels in women of childbearing age should always be checked at the same point in her menstrual cycle. Otherwise, her natural fluctuation that is due to her hormonal balance may be mistaken for an abnormal change in her cholesterol numbers.

♣ The more you understand about cholesterol and what your personal needs and risks are, the better you and your medical provider can determine what cholesterol levels are best for you, because too low can be as risky as too high.

♣ Evidence is mounting that a variety of plant-focused eating patterns are cancer-fighting and promote overall health. These diets include plenty of vegetables, fruit, whole grains, legumes, and nuts, and they also lower risk for type 2 diabetes and cardiovascular disease."

♣ The total number of all the types of cholesterol is less informative than the specific numbers because so much depends on the quality of the laboring cholesterol and the number of housekeepers available to keep our blood clean and free of plaque buildup.

♣ Our body is constantly monitoring and trying to repair itself. It is, therefore, wise for everyone to know as much about how their body uses the foods it consumes. What is Generally Recognized As Safe (GRAS) is *NOT* always be safe for everyone! By blindly trusting the FDA without understanding your body is a risky approach to staying healthy.

References

Bertrais, S. B. (2000). Puberty-associated differences in total cholesterol and triglyceride levels according to sex in French children aged 10–13 years. *Annals for Epidemiology, 10(5)*, 316-323.

Bochem, A. H.-T. (2013). High-density lipoprotein as a source of cholesterol for adrenal steroidogenesis: a study in individuals with low plasma HDL-C. *Journal of Lipid Research, 54(6)*, 1698–1704.

Casteel, B. (2012). *Low cholesterol levels are related to cancer risk.* Retrieved from American College of Cardiology: https://www.acc.org/about-acc/press-releases/2012/03/25/15/15/ldl_cancer

Cordaro, A. A.-E. (2009). *TG/HDL ratio as a surrogate marker for insulin resistance.* Retrieved from European Society of Cardiology: https://www.escardio.org/Journals/E-Journal-of-Cardiology-Practice/Volume-8/TG-HDL-ratio-as-surrogate-marker-for-insulin-resistance

Cox, M. S. (n.d.). *What happens when LDL gets too low?* Retrieved from Sharecare: https://www.sharecare.com/health/cholesterol/what-happens-ldl-cholesterol-low

Derby, C. C. (2009). Lipid changes during the menopause transition in relation to age and weight: The study of women's health across the nation. *Journal of Epidemiology, 169 (11)*, pp. 1352–1361.

Drugs.com. (2018). *Rhabdomyolysis from statins: What's the risk?* Retrieved from Drugs.com: https://www.drugs.com/mcf/rhabdomyolysis-from-statins-what-s-the-risk

Eissa, M. M. (2016). Changes in lipids during puberty. *Journal of Pediatrics, v 170*, pp. 199 - 205.

Elmehdawi, R. (2008). Hypolipidemia: A Word of Caution. *Libyan Journal of Medicine, 3(2)*, 84-90.

Fazio, S. (2013). *Low LDL Syndrome.* Retrieved from Lipids.org: https://www.lipid.org/sites/default/files/14-_fazio-_nla2013_compatibility_mode.pdf

Forones, N. F. (1998). Cholesterolemia in colorectal cancer. *Hepato-gastroenterology, 45(23)*, 1531-1534.

Greenblatt, J. (2011). *Low cholesterol and Its psychological effects: Low Cholesterol is Linked to depression, suicide, and violence.* Retrieved from Psychology Today: https://www.psychologytoday.com/us/blog/the-breakthrough-depression-solution/201106/low-cholesterol-and-its-psychological-effects

Gui D, S. P. (1996). Hypocholesterolemia and risk of death in critically ill surgical patients. *Intensive Care Medicine, 22*, 790 - 794.

Guo X., S. W. (2015). The serum lipid profile of Parkinson's disease patients: a study from China. *Internal Journal of Science 125(11)*, 383 - 844.

Hu, F. M. (2001). Types of dietary fat and risk of coronary heart disease: a critical review. *J Am Coll Nutr.*, 5 -19.

Huang, X. C. (2007). Lower low-density lipid cholesterol levels are associated with Parkinson's disease. *Movement Disorders 22(3)*, 377 381.

Iribarren, C. R. (1995). Serum total cholesterol and mortality. Confounding factors and risk modification in Japanese-American men. *JAMA*, 1926 - 1932.

Khanse, S. (n.d.). *Very-low LDL cholesterol levels: Causes, symptoms, dangers, and treatment.* Retrieved from Health Vigil: Health, medicine, nutrition, and fitness: https://healthvigil.com/low-ldl-cholesterol-levels-causes-symptoms-dangers-treatment/

Lehner, P. (2017). *FDA allows secret, untested chemicals into our food.* Retrieved from Earth Justice, because the earth needs a good lawyer: https://earthjustice.org/blog/2017-june/fda-allows-secret-untested-chemicals-into-our-food

Lemole, G. (2017). *Cholesterol, HDL, and lymphatic clearance of the arterial wall.* Retrieved from Journal of Cardiology and Cardiotherapy: https://juniperpublishers.com/jocct/pdf/JOCCT.MS.ID.555718.pdf

Link, R. (2018). *Niacin foods: Top 15 foods high in niacin & their benefits.* Retrieved from Dr. Axe: Chicken, liver, tuna, turkey, salmon, Sardines, Organic grass-fed beef, Sunflower Seeds, Peanuts. Green Peas, Brown Rice, Mushrooms, Avocado, Sweet Potatoes, Asparagus

Lopez-Jimenez, F. (2018). *Cholesterol level: Can it be too low?* Retrieved from Mayo-Clinic: https://www.mayoclinic.org/diseases-conditions/high-blood-cholesterol/expert-answers/cholesterol-level/faq-20057952

Lotta, L. S. (2016). Association between low-density lipoprotein cholesterol-lowering genetic variants and risk of Type 2 Diabetes. *Journal of Medical Association 316(13)*, 1383 -1891.

Mumford, S. D. (2011). Variations in lipid levels according to menstrual cycle phase: clinical implications. *Clinical Lipidology 6(2)*, 225-234.

NIH. (2010). *Women's cholesterol levels vary with the phase of the menstrual cycle* Bethesda, MD: National Institute of Health.

Orth, M. B. (2012). *Cholesterol: It's regulation and role in Central nervous system disorders.* Retrieved from Creative Commons Attribution: Article ID 292598: https://www.hindawi.com/journals/cholesterol/2012/292598/

Orth, M. B. (2012). *Cholesterol: It's Regulation and Role in Central Nervous System Disorders.* Retrieved from Hindawi, Cholesterol: https://www.hindawi.com/journals/cholesterol/2012/292598/

Pekkanen J1, N. A. (1994). *Changes in serum cholesterol level and mortality: a 30-year follow-up. The Finnish cohorts of the seven countries study.* Retrieved from American Journal of Epidemiology, 139 (2): 155 -165

Rosenberg, A. (2013). *The misery of too low lipids, how they compromise your health and fertility.* Retrieved from Red Mountain Natural Medicine: http://redmountainclinic.com/the-misery-of-low-lipids-how-low-cholesterol-and-low-triglycerides-compromise-your-health-and-fertility/

Schreurs, B. (2010). The Effects of Cholesterol on Learning and Memory. *Neuroscience Biobehavioral Review, Jul, 34(8)*, 1366-1379.

Sullivan, D. (2019). *The difference between VLDL and LDL.* Retrieved from Healthline: https://www.healthline.com/health/vldl-vs-ldl

The Pew Charitable Trusts. (2013). *Fixing oversight of chemicals added to our foods.* Retrieved from PEW: https://www.pewtrusts.org/en/research-and-analysis/reports/2013/11/07/fixing-the-oversight-of-chemicals-added-to-our-food

Tuikkala, P. H. (2010). Serum total cholesterol levels and all-cause mortality in a home-dwelling elderly population: a six-year follow-up. *Scand Journal of Primary Health, 28(2)*, 121 - 127.

Van der Voort, P. G. (2003). HDL-cholesterol level and cortisol response . *Intensive Care Medicine, (29)*, 2199–2203.

Weil, A. (2007). *Low LDL Cholesterol: A Risk For Parkinson's?* Retrieved from Drweil.com: https://www.drweil.com/health-wellness/body-mind-spirit/disease-disorders/low-ldl-cholesterol-a-risk-for-parkinsons/

West R1, B. M. (2008). Better memory functioning associated with higher total and low-density lipoprotein cholesterol levels in very elderly subjects without the apolipoprotein e4 allele. *American Journal of Geriatric Psychiatry. Sep;16(9)*, 781-785.

Wettstein, M. S. (2017). Prognostic Role of Preoperative Serum Lipid levels in patients undergoing radical prostatectomy for clinically localized prostate cancer. *Prostate, 77(5)*, 549 - 556.

Williams, J. (2017). *How to lower dangerously high triglyceride levels.* Retrieved from Renegadehealth: http://renegadehealth.com/blog/2017/03/31/how-to-lower-dangerously-high-triglycerides-levels

Wilson, R. B. (2003). Hypocholesterolemia in sepsis and critically ill or injured patients. *Critical Care, 7(6)*, 413–414.

Wolfson, J. (2017). *The truth about cholesterol and cancer most MD's don't want you to know.* Retrieved from The truth ABout Cancer: Educate, Expose, Erraticate: https://thetruthaboutcancer.com/cholesterol-levels-cancer/

Zhang, Y. X. (2017). Pretreatment direct bilirubin and total cholesterol are significant predictors of overall survival in advanced non-small-cell lung cancer patients with EGFR mutations. *Internal Journal of Cancer, 140(7)*, 1645-1652.

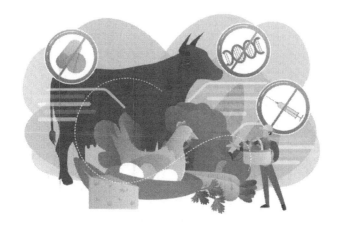

Chapter 7
Food for the American Consumer
Organic vs. Products of Biotechnology

We are what we eat. The food and chemicals that every human and animal ingest affect their health. The foods we choose to eat are major lifestyle choices that can keep us mentally balanced and physically active or cause illnesses, injuries, and premature death.

Diet-related chronic diseases embody the single most significant cause of morbidity and mortality in the USA. Diet-Related chronic diseases afflict 50–65% of our population, whereas most other countries, especially the non-Westernized nations, spend much less on their healthcare, and they live longer with a better quality of life.

Although both scientists and laypeople in the USA often blame a single dietary element as the culprit for their chronic disease (e.g., saturated fat causes heart disease and salt causes high blood pressure), evidence-based research shows that chronic diseases are multifactorial. Chronic ailments are the result of continuous ongoing changes made to our food and environment, all of which disturb our lifestyle choices in a way that causes us to be always adapting. For example, during this last decade, High Fructose Corn syrup (HFCS) has been increasingly added to most processed foods. HFCS is scientifically proven to increase our appetites and cause obesity, which has grown immensely during this past decade. As a result, this particular diet-induced lifestyle change has led to less active with more anxiety in many people, all of which contribute to heart disease and high blood pressure.

In other words, coronary heart disease does not arise simply from excessive saturated fat in the diet, but rather from a complex interaction of multiple nutritional factors directly linked to the excessive consumption of novel industrial-era foods (e.g., plant-based dairy and meat products, refined cereals, refined sugars, refined vegetable oils, trans-fats, transgenetic animal products, and chemical additives). These foods, in turn, not only adversely influence the nutritional value of what we eat but, more importantly, whether our body can use any of the nutrients that come from novel industrial foods. When an innovative industrial food inhibits the absorption or the breakdown of a nutrient into a useable particle, the nutrients are inaccessible and, therefore, not used to contribute to your health. A chemical-additive that is proven to be a hormone-disruptor may be absorbed, but then it causes problems in your hormones. Over time, the problems caused by some novel industrial foods exacerbate chronic diseases of westernized civilization (Cordain, 2010). Many novel processed foods affect our:

- ☺ Glycemic load
- ☺ Fatty acid composition
- ☺ Macronutrient composition
- ☺ Micronutrient density
- ☺ Acid-base balance
- ☺ Sodium-potassium ratio
- ☺ Fiber content

At least ninety different nutrients are needed throughout our life to maintain vitality and regularly restore worn-out cells and tissues. The quality of the foods we consume involves its nutrient content and bioavailability. Remember that bioavailability is the ability of our body to breakdown nutrients and assemble them into compounds our body can use. Food additives and chemical residues can increase or decrease our ability to absorb nutrients. They can also interact with prescribed medication in such a way that it is harmful to that person.

As a consumer, we rely on labels generated by the food industry. We trust that our elected officials implement and update regulations that make sure all foods sold in America are safe to consume and will not cause harm to anyone's health.

Many factors have altered the landscape of our nation over the last 30 or so years, whereas the approval of GMO products has been one of the most influential factors. The production of GMO crops used more than 85 million acres of farmland in the USA, with more added each year (Nolte).

The environmental problems causing chronic illnesses date back much further than 30 years. With the industrial age came the approval of many Products of Biotechnology (POB's) used to control nature. "These include changes and additions to the food we eat, leading to severe nutrient deficiencies, changes in American agriculture and fertility of the soils, more chemicals in the environment, and others" (Onusic, 2013).

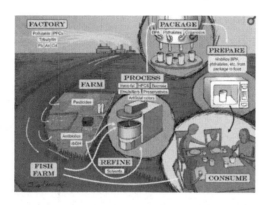

"Compounds are introduced into our food at many stages of the food production process. Waste from factories, including persistent organic pollutants (POPs) and heavy metals (e.g., arsenic, cadmium, and lead), contaminate the water supply. Fish exposed to POB's eat them, and then humans ingest them directly or after further processing. At the farm, these chemicals leach into the crops in the soil, and farmers introduce pesticides to increase crop yield. Animals are fed antibiotics and hormones, which have the potential to be transferred to animal products for human consumption. Crops are then refined to produce the raw ingredient: Insects are removed, organic waste is removed, some products are washed and cooked, and solvents are added to wash away chemicals or isolate desired components. At the processing plant, ingredients are combined to produce the final product. Many of the ingredients used in our food supply have not been tested for their effects on key metabolic pathways. During processing and packaging, food is exposed to plastic-coated pipes and are packaged into plastic containers or plastic-coated cans. Bisphenol A (BPA) is an example of a compound in plastic that can diffuse into food, especially at high temperatures. Next, preparation of the food, especially during heating, can mobilize chemicals in the packaging (e.g., BPA from the baby-bottle into milk during microwaving) or the cookware (e.g., perfluorocarbons (PFCs) from non-stick pans), which can subsequently contaminate the food. Thus, the final food product often contains much more than simply the ingredients added in the large mixer (Figure courtesy of Ian Robert Kleckner)" (Simmons, 2015).

In 1958, the USA government passed legislation to authorize the FDA to regulate all substances added to food. Premarket approval by FDA was required unless the additive is *generally recognized*, amongst qualified experts, to be safe under the conditions of its intended use (GRAS is the acronym for generally recognized as safe). This regulation was sufficient when farmed animals had only their original DNA, were raised in their natural environment, and fed organic food.

This legislation was created before DNA manipulation was used to develop novel animals. Our congress representatives have not updated it since 1958, and therefore neither the FDA or USDA is regulating the safety of novel plants.

As a result, the producers of these novel foods misuse the GRAS legislation by giving (labeling) their novel plant and animal creations organic names, which they are not. For instance, plant-based milk is not the same as animal-based milk, and therefore they do not provide the same nutrients. Furthermore, genetically engineered soy used in many food products in the USA that contains DNA that the general public is unaware of; therefore, those who drink soy milk are not even getting the benefits of organic soy, since at least 94% of all soy sold to the USA consumer is genetically-modified with DNA that Americans are not made aware of.

The reason scientists and food engineers manipulate the DNA (blueprints of life) is to add or remove specific traits in organic plants and animals to produce a particular effect. The effect may be good or bad, depending on whether it improves or harms our health and/or the rest of the environment. Currently, those who profit from novel-foods are responsible for testing its safety with the assumption they perform testing on all of the population, not just those who are very healthy and will not have immediate adverse effects.

Producers of food and additives who want to bypass regulations misuse this loophole in our legislation. By doing so, manufacturers of genetically engineered foods that are considered to be Generally Recognized as Safe (GRAS) are not responsible for the safety of anyone who has unique conditions that make consumption unsafe or for anyone who uses the product in an unintended manner, such as eating more than one-serving within an undetermined amount of time.

In other words, "generally" means that there are some people for whom that food/additive can cause harm. GRAS implies that, in general, healthy people who consume the recommended portions contained in one-serving of one food per day (or longer) should not experience any immediate health problems when they eat or drink that ingredient. It does not guarantee that other additives will not interact in such a way as to cause harm to some people, nor does it mean that eating many foods containing GRAS additives are safe.

Since the ideal treatment for illnesses is prevention, it is ideal that you do not eat any food or additive that can make you sick. Do not consume food that contains harmful ingredients and chemicals and stop eating those that you know are making you sick.

But how do consumers know which additives, processed food, or genetically altered consumables are gradually making them sick in a way that will not be detrimental until years later? Especially when our legislators maintain outdated laws that keep labeling voluntary? Such as the GRAS that should be updated to include FDA regulations for the safety of any plant or animals that is not organic by nature.

How can our medical providers determine when certain foods cause specific symptoms? If the cause is unknown to both the patient/consumer and their medical providers, how can their illness be prevented or treated successfully? The cure is to stop consuming additives and novel foods that make you sick, yet many medical providers will prescribe medication and surgery to reduce the symptoms while the patient continues to consume the ingredients that are causing the symptoms.

Worse yet, in a hasty effort to reduce the symptoms and without knowing the cause, a patient may be instructed to eliminate an entire food group that is otherwise vital to the health and restoration of their body. For example, a patient who has Irritable Bowel Syndrome (IBS), experiences painful bloating and urgent diarrhea after consuming ice cream, yogurt, and cheese. Many of these processed products contain carrageenan, which is known to cause these symptoms (Koon, 2007) (Madden, 2013) (The Cornucopia Institute, 2016). If the cause of the IBS symptoms is the food additive carrageenan, the solution is not to cut out all dairy products, but rather, eliminate all dairy products that contain carrageenan.

The risk associated with eliminating all dairy products includes nutrient deficiencies such as calcium, which builds strong bones and prevents osteoporosis, a vitamin D deficiency, and difficulty absorbing fat-soluble vitamins.

Food is a basic necessity for all forms of life. Apart from nutrition, quality, and cost, the safety of food is of the highest priority. Food-safety requires transparency and traceability. The difference between organic and genetically engineered foods is in how crops are cultivated and farm animals raised, but their differences do not end there. Many foods come from POBs cultivated in a laboratory that requires vast amounts of land to produce their patented cloned and trans-genetic products. They also use chemicals to repel or kill organic life.

Certified organic foods are closely regulated by the USDA. Only farmers and companies that meet the strict standards of organic produce and animal products can put the universal certification emblem on their label, (USDA, nd).

In the USA, genetically engineered foods are not regulated. They are *Generally Recognized As Safe* and therefore do not have any federal legislation that requires disclosure or premarket testing. Instead, they are self-regulated and monitored. Compared to other countries, the regulation of GMOs favors the food industry (Acousta, 2014). GMOs are an economically important component of the biotechnology industry because they own the intellectual property and patents of their human-made foods (Wong, 2016). If they can eliminate the free market of organically grown food, they can control the food industry the way pharmaceuticals control medication. Then we will need an affordable food act!

Since the 1990s, legislators have protected the POB food industry's right to non-disclosure of how food is changing. Labeling foods with one or more applications of POB is voluntary. If a POB food producer worries that consumers won't buy their product if the details about what foreign DNA is added, they do not have to reveal that information on the label. Therefore, consumers may unknowingly consume GM ingredients without their knowledge. If a consumer is allergic to the plant that the foreign DNA came from, that person has no way of knowing they should avoid that innovative processed food.

With the approved technology of gene-manipulation for the past twenty-five years, food scientists have been able to put animal genes into produce, human genes into farm animals, and bacteria-resistant genes into both plants and animals. Since labeling is voluntary, there is no way for the average consumer to know if the food they are buying is genuinely vegetarian or if it contains the same nutrients as its organic counterpart.

For anyone who has allergies, auto-immune deficiencies, or chronic health problems, buying POB foods can be riskier than realized. More than

90% of all food sold to American consumers contains some form of POB technology. Most research surveys claim that as many as 69% of all Americans are unfamiliar with POB food technology but want to learn more.

There have been extreme changes in the American food system over the last twenty-five years. Its effects on Americans have been dramatic. Some of the most influential factors it has had on our society are:

☺ The drop in teen pregnancy, "between 1991 and 2015, the teen pregnancy dropped 64%" (CDC, 2019)

☺ Increased infertility and the use of Assisted Reproductive Technology. "Most childless couples, with a female age under about 43 that are having problems getting pregnant, are considered to be infertile but not sterile" (AFCC, 2017). Causes of infertility range from environmental factors, such as exposure to hormone-disruptor chemicals to physical factors such as obesity, to conditions that prevent the production of sperm or mature eggs, and use of anti-sperm antibodies from human females in seed production (Mahdi, 2011) (NIHCD, 2012)

☺ Increase in the rate of violence (Onusic, 2013)

☺ Learning disabilities, childhood diseases, chronic illnesses, degenerative diseases, cancer, heart disease, diabetes, and obesity in America

It seems that our food industry has sacrificed essential nutrients for the mass production of processed foods. Indeed, it does appear that these changes in our diet, coupled with an increase in the medicalization of the mind and body, and excitotoxic food additives, have provoked an unaffordable health care crisis with appalling consequence. Whereas obesity is not the cure for malnutrition, and obese people are just as likely to be malnourished, it certainly seems like our elected officials for the last 25 years do not have the in incentive to recognize and deal with the factors that have led to our decline in health, increase in infertility and increase in mental disabilities, including those that result in violence.

Crop genetic modification, such as that found in soy and corn, has been gaining popularity, but not without controversy. The main criticisms of POB's are focused on the environmental and health safety of GM crops carrying transgenes. Major environmental concerns include the horizontal transfer of foreign genes into wildlife, the production of "superweeds" that are not killed by conventional doses of herbicides, and the effects of such crops on biodiversity via alterations in the food web. Major health concerns include the potential for allergenicity, infertility, and toxicity of new protein products.

In response to these concerns, the Cartagena Protocol on Biosafety was founded with the goal of controlling the transit and handling of living modified organisms. Several countries have required labeling products with GM ingredients, albeit with different thresholds of tolerance.

The presence of GM maize corn has inadvertently dispersed into the environment. Based on several reports linking genetically modified foods, fragile chromosomal sites in general, and abnormality in the DNA transcription into cancer development in mammals, careful multifaceted investigations of the influence of plant genetic modification on the crop genome and proteome integrity and ultimately the human diet and health are warranted, (Waminal, 2013).

While there are many harmless genetically modified crops, there are others that have the potential to cause irreversible sterility. Genetically modified crops contain the epicyte gene, named for the corporation that created it, Epicyte Pharmaceuticals. Epicyte genes activate a rare class of antibodies that attack sperm. The intended purpose of injecting these genes into soy, corn and other GMO grains was to prevent farmers who bought seeds from specific companies could not save the seeds from their crops and therefore had to buy seeds every year. Now some organic advocates claim, "Scientists have created a GM crop: contraceptive corn. Waiving fields of maize may one day save the world from overpopulation. Researchers have discovered a rare class of human antibodies that attack sperm. By isolating the genes that regulate the manufacture of these antibodies and by putting them in corn plants, the company has created tiny horticultural factories that make contraceptives" (Lewis, 2017).

Infertility is one of the common problems seen in couples of reproductive age. The presence of anti-sperm antibodies in semen and serum are amongst the causes of immune-infertility. This study found that anti-sperm antibodies were found in 62% of vaginal secretions of fertile women and 64% of infertile women. In conclusion, humoral immune response and anti-sperm antibodies may contribute to reproductive failure in couples of reproductive age (Mahdi, 2011).

Frequently, biologists use bacteria to grow human proteins. However, the pharmaceutical company Epicyte decided to put the anti-sperm gene found in sterile human females, into corn. The company says it will not grow this maize near other crops. By isolating the genes that regulate the manufacture of these antibodies and by putting them in corn plants, the company has created horticultural contraceptives. 'We have a hothouse filled with corn plants that make anti-sperm antibodies,' said the Epicyte president. 'We have also created corn plants that make antibodies against the herpes virus, so we should be able to make a plant-based jelly that not only prevents pregnancy but also blocks the spread of sexual disease.' Contraceptive corn is based on research on the rare condition, immune infertility, in which a woman makes antibodies that attack sperm. Essentially, the antibodies are attracted to surface receptors on the sperm. They latch on and make each sperm so heavy it cannot move forward. It just shakes about as if it was doing the lambada' (The Guardian News, 2019).

Essentially, the difference between organic and human-made foods is that organic food is designed by nature to meet our nutritional needs. Organic plants and animals always contain specific genes unique to each species, put there by Mother Nature, whereas human-made foods are created by people that can be influenced by profits and politics. Human-made foods can contain genes and unknown compounds. Fundamentally, organic is the opposite of POB foods. Organic is designed by Mother-Nature to benefit all forms of life on the planet, whereas POB is designed by humans to destroy or control many kinds of nature. In other words, by design, POB is not compatible with organic life.

ORGANIC: MOTHER NATURE'S PLANTS & ANIMALS

Organic food comes from mother nature. Generations of various animals, plants, and micro-organisms continue to exist through reproduction. Only plants and animals of the same species can mate or cross-pollinate. The offspring of both plants and animals contain the genes from their male and female parents, which are passed onto future generations, (Institute of Transformative Bio-Molecules , 2017), (Minako Ueda, 2017). Each form of life has unique traits that help it to survive in its natural environment. For example, some fish naturally have genes that make it endure frigid cold water. Female mammals have genes that make them produce milk after the birth of their offspring.

The word "organic" refers to the way farmers grow and process agricultural products, such as fruits, vegetables, grains, dairy products, and meat. Organic farming practices are designed to meet the following goals (Drugs.com, 2018):

☺ Enhance soil and water quality
☺ Reduce pollution
☺ Provide safe, healthy livestock habitats
☺ Enable natural livestock behavior
☺ Grow grains, fruits, and vegetables that occur naturally in nature
☺ Promote a self-sustaining cycle of resources on a farm

Hybrid plants, also known as cross-breeds, occur in nature when two different varieties of the same species of plants cross-pollinate to form offspring. The outcome may make it more adaptable to the environment, and sometimes it tastes better. Hybrid strains can evolve into a new variety that will produce fertile seeds that may be a combination of both parents or revert back to one or the other parents' original traits. A test to determine whether an organic-plants is truly organic is to save seeds from a fruit or vegetable and plant them in organic soil. If they grow, they have not been genetically altered with genes from a totally different species of life.

Mother Nature freely replenishes plants and animals without government interventions or industrial monopolies. Fertile organic seeds from plants grow the same produce planted in natural soil and can be saved to plant future crops without violating seed and soil patents. This is because no one owns the intellectual property rights for Mother Nature's creation.

The next time you eat a delicious organic tomato, try saving some of the seeds from one of the jelly-like grooves and put them in organic soil. Each seed will grow into a tomato plant that produces multiple tomatoes with the same DNA and RNA as the original tomato, and therefore it will also provide you with the same nutrients. All this can come from the freely saved seeds.

All living things are made up of macro and micro molecules: Nucleic acids, lipids, proteins, and carbohydrates. In nature, all forms of life contain distinctive characteristics that are regarded as unchangeable. Nucleic acids are *species-specific*. Each DNA and RNA module are aligned with matching pairs. The passing of similar genes from generation to generation is Mother

Nature's guarantee that two organic parents will always produce the same species.

When plants and animals are used for food, they always contain the same nutrients, because their genes consistently carry the same genetic information. In other words, every variety of organic apples will always provide the same basic nutrients; hence, the old saying "an apple a day will keep the doctor away," is a wise old adage that promotes healthy dietary choices. All varieties of organic apples provide many nutrients such as vitamins A and C, iron, protein, and their skin are rich in insoluble fiber that is valuable to our microbiota.

Predictably, all forms of organic life consume nutrients obtained from other organic life. When and if the environment changes, each living thing must adapt to those changes in order to survive, which leads to some natural DNA instructional changes. This is Mother Nature's way of helping life to survive. Each form of life has its own set life-cycle and built into nature are ways to remove the dead to make way for new life. Mother Nature makes all of her products biodegradable.

Within various environmental settings, plants and animals help each other survive. One personal example is in my garden. I had a citronella plant by my house that was in poor health and ready to die. In my garden, my tomato plants were thriving, but nothing to brag about. Somehow, either a bird or maybe a strong wind blew a tomato seed into the pot of my citronella plant. The organic tomato plant grew large and full of old fashion tasty tomatoes. As for the citronella plant, it revived itself into a thick luscious plant full of rich lemony smelling oil.

Mother nature has a way of healing itself when left to do so. The natural progression of produce continues to mature until they are ripe and then begin to decompose by micro-organisms that not only thrive on the fruit but keep the planet clean by breaking them down into elements the earth can recycle. Within the digestive system, our gut's eco-system /microbiota helps further Breakdown nutrients for us to use. All forms of life use nutrients to manufacture their own hormones, enzymes, and other supplies needed to sustain life.

The way plants and animals interact in the environment sustains Mother Nature's ecosystem. Humans were a part of this cycle. Homemakers, chefs, and bakers use organic plants and animals to create meals for family, friends, and themselves.

Organic produce, meat, and dairy products are essential for the creation of organic foods and beverages, which are essential to the American economy.

Land is used by farmers to grow organic life. All humans need food to survive. Organic life is a natural resource. A country with no natural resources has nothing to offer the world and cannot sustain itself.

Organic food is grown without the use of synthetic pesticides, bioengineered genes (GMOs), petroleum-based fertilizers, and sewage sludge-based fertilizers. Organic livestock raised for meat, eggs, and dairy products must have access to the outdoors and be given organic feed. They are not given any antibiotics or growth hormones.

Organic crop farming materials or practices may include (Drugs.com, 2018):

☺ Plant waste left on fields (green manure), livestock manure or compost to improve soil quality
☺ Plant rotation to preserve soil quality and to interrupt cycles of pests or disease
☺ Cover crops that prevent erosion when parcels of land are not in use and to plow into soil for improving soil quality
☺ Mulch to control weeds
☺ Predatory insects or insect traps to control pests
☺ Certain natural pesticides and a few synthetic pesticides approved for organic farming used rarely and only as a last resort in coordination with a USDA organic certifying agent

Organic farming practices for livestock include (Drugs.com, 2018):

☺ Healthy living conditions and access to the outdoors
☺ Pasture feeding for at least 30 percent of livestock's nutritional needs during the grazing season
☺ Organic foods for animals
☺ Vaccinations

The benefits of organic foods are that they are predictably rich in nutrients and antioxidants; they consistently contain only genes natural to those forms of life. Since they have no contact with laboratory chemicals, people with allergy to foods or preservatives often feel better when they eat only organic foods. People allergic to the GMO form of produce and animal products are not necessarily allergic to the original organic form, because cross-contamination and the use of foreign genes are not added to organic products.

"There is a growing body of evidence that shows some potential health benefits of organic foods when compared with conventionally grown foods. While these studies have shown differences in the food, there is limited information to draw conclusions about how these differences translate into overall health benefits. Potential benefits are (Drugs.com, 2018):

☺ **Nutrients -** Studies have shown small to moderate increases in some nutrients in organic produce. The best evidence of a significant increase is in certain types of flavonoids, which have antioxidant properties.

☺ **Omega-3 fatty acids -** The feeding requirements for organic livestock farming, such as the primary use of grass and alfalfa for cattle, result in generally higher levels of omega-3 fatty acids, a kind of fat that is more heart-healthy than other fats. These higher omega-3 fatty acids are found in organic meats, dairy, and eggs.

☺ **Toxic metal -** Cadmium is a toxic chemical naturally found in soils and absorbed by plants. Studies have shown significantly lower cadmium levels in organic grains, but not fruits and vegetables, when compared with conventionally grown crops. The lower cadmium levels in organic grains may be related to the ban on synthetic fertilizers in organic farming.

☺ **Pesticide residue -** Compared with conventionally grown produce, organically grown produce has lower detectable levels of pesticide residue. Organic produce may have residue because of pesticides approved for organic farming or because of airborne pesticides from conventional farms. The difference in health outcomes is unclear because of safety regulations for maximum levels of residue allowed on conventional produce.

☺ **Bacteria -** Meats produced conventionally may have a higher occurrence of bacteria resistant to antibiotic treatment. The overall risk of bacterial contamination of organic foods is the same as conventional foods.

This is one reason why most nations are very vigilant in protecting its organic food supply. At least 130 nations have signed an agreement that prevents the cultivation and/or sale of genetically engineered foods using biotechnology (POB) prior to proof of safety. The development of this safety standard began in the 1970s when biotechnology began genetic experimentation. It was not until America deregulated the cultivation and sale of POB foods in 1994 that the World Health organization finalize the agreement known as the Cartagena Act. In 2003, these protocols were finalized and enacted internationally. American elected officials have since refused to sign this agreement.

This international agreement uses precautionary principles prior to the use or sale of POB foods and medications. It empowers the nations that sign onto this agreement, to ban any POB products that they determined to be unsafe to humans and/or their environment. For example, the Cartagena Acts protect their country's right to demand all GMO foods be accurately labeled and ban imports of GMO food and medicines if they feel there is sufficient scientific evidence proving the product is unsafe and may harm its citizens or their environment. It also requires exporters to label shipments containing genetically altered commodities such as soy, corn, and cotton. This means the American food industries that exercise their right not to label GMO ingredients when selling their products in America must use a different packaging label when selling to the more than 130 nations that require it.

If our American elected officials had signed the Cartagena Act, the cultivation and sale of POB foods would be limited to only those products proven to be safe. Also, labeling would become mandatory.

In America, organic food is produced by methods that comply with the standards of organic farming. Standards vary worldwide. Essentially, organic farming protects the ecological balance of life and preserves biodiversity. Organizations regulating organic products restrict the use of certain pesticides and fertilizers in the farming methods used to produce such products. Organic foods are not processed using irradiation, industrial solvents, or synthetic food additives.

In the 21st century, the European Union, the United States, Canada, Mexico, Japan, and many other countries require producers to obtain special certification to market their food as *organic*. Selling food with an organic label is regulated by governmental food safety authorities, such as the National Organic Program of the US Department of Agriculture (USDA) and the European Commission (EC).

From an environmental perspective, fertilizing, overproduction, and the use of pesticides in conventional (non-organic) farming harms the ecosystems, biodiversity, groundwater, and drinking water supplies. These environmental and health issues are intended to be minimized or avoided in organic farming.

For centuries farmers rotated crops, fertilized their fields with manure from organically fed farm animals, and composted old plants to keep their soil rich in nutrients that ultimately help their crops grow bigger and tastier. Manure from organic cows, horses, chickens, goats, and sheep contain cellulose decomposing bacteria along with undigested active digestive enzymes. These animals do not carry the same diseases as humans; therefore, their manure does not infect soil with diseases known to harm humans. Instead, the undigested enzymes contribute to faster heating of the manure, which accelerates the decomposition of organic materials by the soil microorganisms. The end result of better decomposition of organic material is faster nutrient release to crops that is safe to humans and the rest of the environment (Better gardening, 2019).

Farmers use many acres of land for their livestock to graze on natural grass and grains. Poultry scratched the land to find bugs and worms. Even seafood had relied on natural sea flora for survival. Whatever these animals consume affects the quality of their bodies, which then impacts the quality of the food they produce. Nutrient-rich foods help build their life-sustaining enzymes and hormones, which then produce eggs and milk intended for the production of new life.

In 1990, Congress passed the Organic Foods Production Act (OFPA). OFPA mandated the USDA to set forth a national standard for organic food and fiber production. This department continues to be responsible for implementing, monitoring, and explaining this law to producers, handlers, and certifiers. A copy of this handbook can be downloaded from the USDA website for OFPA (USDA, nd).

While organic farming has not changed very much in the past thirty years, labeling a product "organic" mandates by law that food has been grown following the federal guidelines of the Organic Foods Production Act. This national standard requires all organic producers who sell over $5,000 annually in agricultural products and want to label their product "organic" must be certified by a USDA-accredited agency. Companies that process organic food must also be certified.

Any farms or handling operations with less than $5,000 a year in organic agricultural products are exempt from certification. Those producers may label their products organic if they follow the standards, but they are prohibited from displaying the USDA Organic Seal, (SARE, ND), (Gold, 2007, 2018).

The use of herbicides, fungicides, and other chemicals are banned in organic produce.

One of the Non-GMO Project certification requirements is, "To be a certified organic producer, you have to go through three crop cycles in order to get the land certified. You can then do non-GMO next year" (Porterfield, 2016). This assures that the land used to grow organic crops is free of pesticides and chemicals, and the seeds only contain organic genes.

Demand for organic foods is driven by consumer concerns for personal health and the environment. Claims that "organic food tastes better" is consumer preference; the difference may be in the freshness of farmed foods.

Since 1994, here has been extensive international evidence-based-research in the scientific and medical literature to support claims that organic food is safer and healthier to eat than many POB foods. Their differences in the nutrient contents of organic versus conventionally produced food depend on the type of POB food production. For instance, when DNA from seafood, E-coli bacterium, and the antibiotic Kanamycin was injected into the Flavr Savr tomato, those tomatoes most certainly contained a different nutrient value than the organic tomato that did not contain those genes.

I have also been told by multiple people that organic food is too expensive. I know from personal experience that growing produce can be very cheap once your garden has been established. Organic seeds can be saved for even more savings, but even buying organic seeds is cost-effective. One packet of organic lettuce seeds costs $5.00 and produces over 250 heads of lettuce. Each $5.00 investment in packets of tomato or other produce seeds can produce hundreds of dollars in savings.

On the other hand, for those not inclined to have a garden, shop around. Recently my partner purchased two dozen cage-free non-GMO and organic certified eggs at a local supermarket. He paid $5.99 per dozen eggs plus $6.99 for a gallon of organically certified milk. When I realized this, I took him to a different store known to sell only organic products. There, the exact same brand of cage-free non-GMO and certified eggs cost $2.59 per dozen, and a gallon of organically certified milk was $4.99. Our local general supermarket charged him $8.80 more for two certified organic products than another store was charging on the same day.

The lesson learned here is that some stores falsely inflate organic prices, which makes them appear too expensive for a large family. My guess is that these supermarkets either do so to increase their profits, or they receive incentives from POB food producers (organic competitors) to trick consumers into buying non-organic foods.

Another lesson learned from recent years of experience arose from my desire to have a garden again. I dreamed of the large garden I had back in the 1970s until 1996. Every seed produced tasty fruits and vegetables in the same soil I used all those years. Each spring, I tilled the soil, planted seeds, and waited for them to grow. There were weeds, but mom was my weed controller. She was great!

Every year I grew a large variety of beans, berries, tomatoes, and much more in quantities sufficient enough to feed my family and friends with enough left over to can and freeze for a full winter's supply of these crops. Only the first few years required extensive work to set it up. Once in place, very little needed to be done to keep it going.

When I moved out of state, I tried to start a new garden, but this time I bought most of the dirt I put into raised-beds. I bought plants instead of seeds to get a head start. Those plants grew lush with greenery but produced very few crops that were bland. Hardly worth the effort of growing them. Worse yet, the few seeds I was able to save either did not sprout, or they grew something totally different.

I was working as a nurse at the time and had little time to figure out why I lost my ability to grow enough vegetables to feed myself, let alone a family. Only in the last three years have I taken up this hobby again. The first year I bought soil, plants, and a few seeds that all pretty much failed to produce nice crops. As I became more aware of POBs, I decided to collect organic soil from each state where I traveled by digging up buckets of soil to bring home. I also used only organic soils with no chemicals added when purchased from the store. I then purchased all my seeds from Seed Exchange, which sells organic seeds. Much to my amazement and that of my friends, my garden once again flourished.

When I first started this garden, many neighbors warned me that crops could not grow this close to the beach, but I proved them wrong! I have a 20' x 15' fenced-in garden that produced plenty of fresh organic tomatoes, lettuce, beans, herbs, and a variety of other crops we enjoy year-round. I use organic flowers and plants to detract bugs and the fence to keep my dogs out, because, apparently, they too love fresh organic tomatoes and lettuce.

In general, people eat organic food for many reasons. Those who eat an organic diet are exposed to fewer disease-causing pesticides, and organic farming is more sustainable and better for the environment.

Food safety tips (Drugs.com, 2018):

Whether you go totally organic or opt to mix conventional and organic foods, be sure to keep these tips in mind:

☺ **Select a variety of foods from a variety of sources.** This will give you a better mix of nutrients and reduce your likelihood of exposure to a single pesticide.

☺ **Buy fruits and vegetables in season when possible.** To get the freshest produce, ask your grocer what is in season or buy food from your local farmers market.

☺ **Read food labels carefully.** Just because a product says it's organic or contains organic ingredients does not necessarily mean it's a healthier alternative. Some organic products may still be high in sugar, salt, fat, or calories.

☺ **Wash and scrub fresh fruits and vegetables thoroughly under running water.** Washing helps remove dirt, bacteria, and traces of chemicals from the surface of fruits and vegetables, but not all pesticide residues can be removed by washing. Discarding outer leaves of leafy vegetables can reduce contaminants. Peeling fruits and vegetables can remove contaminants but may also reduce nutrients.

PRODUCTS OF BIOTECHNOLOGY (POB) FOODS

POB foods do not occur naturally in nature. POB plants and animals are created in a laboratory where organic life is altered. Fundamentally, POBs are the opposite of organic life in that they are manmade plants and animals. Methods to control loss of crops and increase productivity for both agriculture and animal farmers have been used for many centuries, but genetic alterations have only come about in the last seventy years and were not approved for food consumption until 1994. Unfortunately, many manmade compounds in our food supply are added deliberately to enhance production regardless of their impact on nutrition. For example, pesticides are used to ward off insects during farming; BPA is a durable, clear plastic that has ideal properties for making bottles and coating cans; and mono- and diglycerides are added to emulsify the fat and water in foods to achieve a favorable texture (Simmons, 2015).

Materials or practices not permitted in organic farming, but can be used in POB production include (Drugs.com, 2018):

☺ Synthetic fertilizers to add nutrients to the soil
☺ Human sewage sludge as fertilizer
☺ Synthetic pesticides for pest control
☺ Irradiation to preserve food or to eliminate disease or pests
☺ Use of genetic engineering to improve disease or pest resistance or to improve crop yields
☺ Antibiotics or growth hormones for livestock

Their products are not bred in traditional forms that require male-female reproduction. Instead, scientists apply biotechnological methods created in a laboratory that is intended to control and/or change organic life. By adding or removing specific genes, scientists can add unnatural traits that resist diseases and drought. Scientists can remove features that attract pests so that their products repel them. Food engineers are also able to add features that harm pests physically, chemically, or biologically by interfering with their metabolism, reproduction, and/or behavior (EPA, 2018).

Mother Nature's resources are altered to create products that resemble typical organic food but changed enough to be patented and sold for profit (Hauck, 2014). The food industry, including its scientists and engineers, claims that the goal of their products is to reduce world hunger someday and improve global health. Many POB gardening products imply they will increase production. My personal experience with POB foods and gardening have not supported this, but according to the Borgen Project (McComb, 2016):

> "GMOs undergo rigorous testing (a period ranging from five to eight years) conducted by the U.S. Environmental Protection Agency, U.S. Department of Agriculture, and the Food and Drug Administration to make sure the genetically modified food is safe for human consumption. Currently, there is no legislation requiring food packagers to label the genetically modified food that sits on supermarket shelves.
>
> GMOs have the potential to help solve food production issues in the future, making a dent in the fight against global poverty. Yet it is important to recognize the reality of and work to address the downsides, as the introduction of GMO crops (large, industrialized yields) to a country's economy could change local farming practices (smaller, local yields), may dominate their food markets, can harm the environment through the required pesticides and can result in large-scale monocultures."

In the meantime, millions of acres of farmland and government money are used for the production of POB. For example, one "four-year project, which was supported by various government agencies, including $30 million from the National Science Foundation," used thousands of acres of farmland and millions of tons of water to produce genetically altered corn maize (Harmon, 2009). For more than a generation now, research has consistently found GMO corn used for human consumption to cause obesity, diabetes, resistance to the hormone leptin, malnutrition, and a host of other chronic human diseases (Shapiro, 2008). It also found that farmed-fish fed GMO corn grew twice as fast in half the time, (Center for Food Safety, 2018) and passed that trait on to its consumers-- making us fat (Foss, 2012), sterile and impotent, (Hayden, 2011). Disposal of trans-genetic, cloned, and GMO products are treated like biohazard waste, including any bedding used during the lifecycle of these animals, and must be carefully contained and incinerated to prevent damage to any organic life and the environment (EHS, 2017) (Woodson, 2004).

Multiple countries ban all GMO foods while others only ban their cultivation; those countries allow GMO grains that have been milled and, therefore, cannot leak into their environment (GMO FAQ, 2018).

Being that POB's are the intellectual property of the food industry, the price of these foods is controlled by those who own their patents (Acousta,

2014) (Wong, 2016). Of equal concern, "the truth is, we don't know enough about GMOs to deem them safe for human consumption. There is a multitude of credible scientific studies that clearly demonstrate why GMO's should not be consumed, and more are emerging every year" (Walia, 2014). Fundamentally, scientifically engineered foods are empowering the food industry to control the supply and demand of food in much the same way that the pharmaceutical industry controls the availability and price of medications.

One particular pollutant to the planet that has since been banned is Poly-Chlorinated Biphenyls (PCB), which is a class of manmade "organic" chemicals. Each PCB molecule contains two phenyl rings. A phenyl ring is a ring of 6 carbon atoms to which hydrogen atoms are attached. In PCBs, chlorine atoms replace some of these hydrogen atoms (Greenfacts.org, 2019).

This scientifically engineered contaminant, PCBs, is worth mentioning at this point, because of its ongoing existence in the environment has consequences on the additional genetically engineered food products. PCBs were created in 1929, leading to widespread industrial use. By the time they were banned in 1977, one chemical company had already started selling another toxic chemical containing glyphosates and dicamba called Roundup, while PCBs continued to contaminate our air, land, and water. In addition to the introduction of these other chemicals, PCB's are in a classification known as Persistent Organic Pollutants, because they remain in the environment (WDF, Unk.) (Foster, 2016) (WDHS, 2018).

The U.S. Environmental Protection Agency (EPA) determined that PCBs cause cancer in all animals (EPA, 1999). Many rivers and buildings, including schools, parks, farmland, and other sites are contaminated with PCBs. There has been contamination of food supplies with the substances (WDF, Unk.) (EPA, 1999). Some of the many toxic effects of PCBs are neurotoxicity and endocrine disruption, caused by blocking thyroid system functions (Boas, 2006).

Given the previous environmental contaminants such as PCB's from 1930 through 1977, the inception of glyphosate and dicamba (Roundup) in 1975, causes additional harm to our environment, (Bonn, 2005), (Richard, 2005). It is alarming to realize government officials since 1994 have allowed unregulated and unlabeled genetical alterations made to our food (Foster, 2016). Is there any confusion as to why chronic illnesses, especially childhood diseases over the last two decades has risen? (GMO Science, 2015) (Owens K. F., 2010).

"About 43% of US children (~14 million out of 32 million) have at least 1 of 20 different chronic health conditions (Bethell, 2011). Even more worrisome is that the incidence rates of the following diseases and conditions have shown significant increases in the last 20 years, but with no clear explanations: Cancer (Linabery, 2008), asthma and allergies (Radhakrishnan, 2014), including allergies requiring hospitalization (Devereux, 2006), type 1 diabetes (Lipman, 2013), inflammatory bowel disease (Malaty, 2010), behavioral and learning disabilities (Halfon, 2012), and (although it is somewhat debated) autism spectrum disorder (Hertz-Picciotto, 2009)" (GMO Science, 2015).

Had POB's been known to be safe and healthy, their induction to our food supply would have been broadcasted all over the news media and included in education, but sadly this was not the case. Instead of warning Americans, many lawmakers chose to pass laws to help the food industry covertly sell POB's to consumers.

The demand and cost of medical care have since increased from a national cost of $8.5 billion at roughly $3,000 per American annually in 1994 to $4 trillion at the cost of about $12,000 per American (Amedeo, 2018). Many researchers attribute this increase to the use of POB foods, unbeknownst to most American consumers. Additives and contaminant residues are directly linked to the rise in chronic illnesses in the USA. In fact, America used to be a world leader in healthcare but has fallen far behind other nations in quality and outcomes (Olsen, 2016).

The Institute for Health Metrics and Evaluation and reported by Bloomberg shows that the U.S. is expected to fall in global life expectancy rankings over the next few decades. In 2016, the U.S. ranked 43rd among 195 nations, with an average life expectancy of 78.7 years. If nothing changes, this trend is expected to keep spiraling downward to 64th by 2040 (Weiner, 2018) with the cost of medical care is anticipated to keep rising.

Not all POB's are to blame for the decline in health and an increase in medical care. Many processed foods are safe to consume when consumed in recommended serving sizes and are minimally used with a diet mostly of organic foods. Health problems occur when additives with known side-effects are consumed in multiple foods and large serving sizes. Hence, consumers must take responsibility to know what they are eating and drinking and making sure they are not ingesting amounts that cause their own illnesses.

There are a variety of scientific methods used by the POB food industry to control and change Mother Nature's organic food sources. The most common POB food technologies are:

☺ Genetically Modified Organisms (GMO)
☺ Genetic Use Restriction Technologies (GURT)
☺ Biocides: Pesticides, Herbicides, Fungicides, and Rodenticides
☺ Fortified with Food Additives, Preservatives, and Chemicals
☺ Cloned, Trans-genetic & Test-tube Meats
☺ Functional Foods

GENETICALLY MODIFIED ORGANISMS (GMO) & TRANS GENETIC ANIMALS

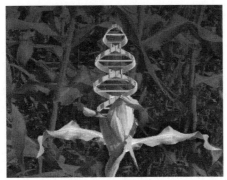

Food engineers extract DNA that is unique to particular plants, animals, or microbes and inject them into the DNA of different plants and animals to create their own individual forms of life. These man-made crops and creatures cannot reproduce themselves; therefore, the food industry controls its production.

By simply swapping a strand of DNA molecules in a cow, with human DNA, food engineers have made cows that produce human milk. By adding some growth hormones, they increase milk production, and by sprinkling in a few bacteria genes further down the chromosome chain, they prevent mastitis caused by the irritation of human milk in the cow's udders. Cows fortified with human genes also produce human plasma for medical treatments (Ormandy, 2011).

Over the last twenty-five years, there has been a sharp increase in chronic illnesses, especially global diabetes. When the artificial sweetener HFCS was introduced into the American food supply, children for the first time began getting type II diabetes, and obesity rates soared. Since there are no enzymes in the human body to digest HFCS, it has to be metabolized by the liver. As a result, the pancreas cannot release insulin the way it usually does for organic sugar, so fructose converts to fat more readily than any other sugar. An overworked liver produces significantly more uric acid, multiplying the risk for heart disease (Highfructosecornsyrup.org, 2009).

In response to HFCS being a leading cause of diabetes, scientists are now alerting consumers that insulin will be in short supply by 2030, due to the rise in childhood and adult diabetes (Lapidus, 2018). Yet, large amounts of GMO sugar-additives continue to be a significant additive in most processed foods. For scientists and our elected officials, the solution lies with more unregulated POBs such as cultivating pigs with human genes to manufacture human insulin and human organs for human transplants (Tonti-Filippini, 2001), instead of a logical and less costly solution, such as banning the additives that are causing the health problems like other countries have.

Genetically engineered plants, animals, bacteria, and viruses, can perform many amazing things, all without the consumers' knowledge. Examples of GMO foods available to the American consumer are:

- ✓ GMO Bananas that contain vaccines and birth control (Moss, 2010).

- ✓ GMO Peanut Butter: natural peanut oils substituted with GMO grain oils, GMO soy, and maize corn reduce the nutritional value (Segedie, 2019) while increasing bulk for profit.

- ✓ GMO Corn made into HFCS; A beverage analyst estimated that by switching to HFCS soda manufactures gained a cost advantage of USD 70 million a year (Highfructosecornsyrup.org, 2009).

- ✓ GMO Golden Rice fortified with vitamin A from daffodils (Dubock, 2014) (Everding, 2016)

- ✓ Tomatoes contained genes from seafood, E-coli bacteria, and the antibiotic-resistant protein from the antibiotic Kanamycin to extend shelf life (Flanders, 2018).

- ✓ Aqua Advantage salmon is wild-caught salmon injected with Chinook-salmon growth hormones and eelpout DNA, (Center for Food Safety, 2018), (Greger, 2012).

✓ GMO Grains are used to produce many dietary oils at a reduced cost

✓ Farm animals fed GMO grains, including grains made from cow manure (Majda, 2014).

✓ GMO soy is used to make the Impossible burger look and allegedly taste like a real burger. It even bleeds plant-based imitation blood when bitten into (Yu, 2018).

Food scientists and engineers can turn genes on or off in many forms of organic life. The reasons for doing so can be anything from increasing our appetites, so we consume more food, to increase the production of crops. Scientists can even manipulate the way food is digested and stored or eliminated (Main, 2012), or induce infertility that may control specific populations (Swanson, 2013). A broad group of scientists and scholars challenge the safety of these unregulated and untested alterations to our food (Hilbeck, 2015).

Compared to wild freshwater fish and seafood that live off the flora in lakes, rivers, and the ocean, farmed fish are fed GMO grains that are designed to increase appetites and store fat, so they grow larger than their wild counterparts (Main, 2012). For instance, many brands of farmed salmon fed GMO corn and other grains, designed to stimulate their appetites, made them grow as much as 1000% larger. One study showed their intestines had altered microbiota, making them less able to digest proteins. It also caused them to store more fat and changed their immune systems. Blood samples also showed these changes in their blood (Foss, 2012).

Aqua Advantage salmon are genetically altered with from eel-pout, an ocean fish. By exchanging specific DNA, this increases the salmon growth hormone to make it grow fatter faster. By reaching their slaughter size quicker, it reduces the consumption of GMO grains by 25%, which is a big saving to the producer (Goodman, 2015). Unfortunately, those abnormal genes are then passed onto consumers, making some people grow fatter faster (Foss, 2012).

Food-Scientists can take genes from plants that are naturally drought resistant and inject them into an organic vegetable to reduce their dependency on water. They also insert genes that produce resistance to fungus and bacteria. This extends their shelf life indefinitely because microorganisms that typically breakdown these foods are repelled. Consequently, those resistant genes can also resist the healthy microbiota in the gut of humans, pets, and wildlife, which usually breakdown these foods into usable nutrients.

The first GMO produce sold to Americans in 1996 was the Flavr Savr tomato. These tomatoes looked like organic tomatoes. As such, consumers were not aware; these tomatoes contained genes from E-coli bacteria, Kanamycin antibiotic, and cold-water seafood. They all matured at the same time, were the same size with the exact same color and tough skin to make picking more manageable, but their genetic makeup was not the same as organic tomatoes, and therefore, their nutrient value was different.

Because consumers were not made aware of the new DNA injected into the Flavr Savr tomato, those with autoimmune deficiencies or allergies to seafood had no way of knowing they should avoid these tomatoes. Medical professionals were not made aware either; therefore, new chronic conditions with unknown origins became a medical mystery that inevitably increased the cost and demand for medical attention with no way of knowing the cause.

Since then, many more GMO foods and additives have been added to American foods. The impossible burger looks so real that someone allergic to GMO soy may mistakenly consume a soy-burger and then have a severe allergic reaction. Both the patient and their medical provider will be baffled when the patient insists they have not consumed any soy. And one must wonder, will that medical provider instruct that person to stop eating all beef?

Produce can have vaccines and genes injected that do not decompose through digestion in the human body. Instead, it blends into the consumer's own DNA, making them resistant to certain antibiotics while rendering others infertile (Key, 2008) (Moss, 2010) (The Guardian, 2018). Many studies prove that DNA and RNA from GMO foods are passed on to the consumer (Key, 2008).

Extensive research in China found that genes injected into food survive digestion and plays a role in causing human diseases, including cancer, Alzheimer's, Attention Deficit Hyperactivity Disorders, heart disease, high cholesterol, and diabetes. They usually function by turning down or shutting down specific natural genes that typically combat diseases. This indicates that in addition to the vitamins, proteins, fats, and carbs we get from the foods we eat, we are also consuming gene regulators as designated by the food industry and regulated by government agencies (Zhang, 2012) (Le Vaux, 2012), (GMO Awareness, 2014). The old saying, an apple a day will keep the doctor away, may no longer be true, because not all apples in the supermarket are created equal. In fact, some may actually cause severe reactions.

As Americans are becoming more aware of POB products, many still do not understand that GMO crops are not the same as Nature's organic produce. When genes from animals, seafood, bacteria, and plant life are added or removed from a fruit, vegetable, or animal product, it no longer contains the same nutrients as its organic counterpart. Remember how DNA and RNA manage and replicate every cell in the body. GMO products have different and unique information in their genes that can get into our cells.

What scientists have come to appreciate is the genetic material of the plants and animals we consume do have the ability to alter the behavior of the enzyme and its effects on nutrients in our bodies. Since DNA and RNA originate from the genetic material in a cell, the raw-genes we are exposed to when eating GMO food can mix with our own genes, (Banks Nutrition, 2012). Those who are strict vegan should also be aware that some produce many contain genes from animals and seafood.

For American consumers to make better-informed choices that promote health and reduce the need for medical interventions, we need more information and better regulation of our food and environment. common sense tells us that a self-regulated industry that is profiting from overconsumption of food is not going to fix the problems they created, let alone admit to them.

Several individuals who previously held high-ranking positions in FDA and the Department of Health and Human Services (HHS) reported that in the last 25 years, cuts to spending on the FDA has increasingly put the FDA at risk of being unable to adequately fulfill the many statutory responsibilities that Congress used to assign it. While the call for more resources has been heard by our Congress, "the United States continues to spend significantly more on health care than any other nation. In 2006, our health care expenditure was more than twice the average of 29 other developed countries. We have one of the fastest growth rates in health spending, tripling our expenditures since 1990, yet the average life expectancy in the United States is far below many other nations that spend far less on health care each year" (CDC, 2009).

According to one congressional report, "There is a growing debate about whether the Food and Drug Administration (FDA) has the ability to accomplish its mission with the resources provided by congressional appropriations. FDA plays a central role in protecting public health in the United States by regulating most of the food supply that affects American lives on a daily basis. A 2006 report on by the Institute of Medicine (IOM) reported their findings that indicated the FDA lacks the resources necessary to accomplish its complex mission, let alone its position to meet future challenges. There is no doubt the FDA is severely underfunded" (Members and Committee of Congress, 2008).

There is no doubt that Americans want healthy food that has been thoroughly tested for safety before sold to us, and all agree the FDA, USDA, and EPA must be adequately funded to do so, but must also be assigned full authority to do their jobs right.

Genetic Use Restriction Technologies (GURT)

GURT is called the terminator or suicide seeds because they contain Epicyte genes (human anti-sperm) that make them unable to produce offspring (Lewis, 2017), (Waminal, 2013). Gurt seeds produce only one generation of large abundant infertile crops.

> "The ultimate seeds of suicide are patented technology to create sterile seeds. Called *Terminator technology* by the media, sterile seed technology is a type of Gene Use Restriction Technology, GRUT, in which seed produced by a crop will not grow. Crops will not produce viable offspring seeds, nor will it produce viable seeds with its specific genes switched off" (Shiva, 2018).

They are also bred to be Herbicide Tolerant (HT). These plants are bred for resistance to herbicides such as glyphosate and dicamba, which are used by farmers' ability to control weeds and enhances crop yields. HT crops can be sprayed with herbicides without being harmed, while all other plants are killed. This allows farmers to spray their crops with these specific herbicides without risking harm to their crops. Among the crops with these traits are corn, cotton, canola, soybeans, sugar beets, and alfalfa (Genetic Literacy Program, 2016).

Farmers who grow these crops must purchase the seeds and herbicide from the manufacturer (who owns the patent for those seeds) each year. This is a concern for farmers and gardeners who seed-save and grow organic crops because these crops can cross-pollinate with organic crops in nearby areas, causing those plants to become sterile and die (Convention on Biodiversity, 1999). This is one key reason why many countries that ban the cultivation of GURT and GMO seeds but allow GMO ingredients in processed foods. They require these grains to be "milled" and crushed prior to entering their country, so GMO grains cannot accidentally cross-pollinate with their organic plants.

The herbicide Roundup contains two harsh chemicals: Glyphosate and dicamba. Together they disrupt the formation of digestive enzymes in all forms of organic plant life, which causes starvation and death (Bonn, 2005),

(Haefs R, 2002). The leading brand of GURT seeds are Roundup Ready seeds; these are seeds that have the antidote for Roundup built into their DNA. Therefore, the enzymes in their plants are resistant to glyphosates and dicamba (Roundup). Their seeds and crops can be sprayed with Roundup many times throughout the growing season and still grow, while all other plant life dies.

Together, dicamba and glyphosate herbicides kill all forms of plant life except those that contain the antidote for Roundup. Crops grown from seeds that are Roundup ready can be sprayed many times to kill off all other forms of plant life, and those crops will flourish, even as this herbicide seeps into the earth's aqua-filter and drains off into nearby waterways, (NPIC, 2012). One of the most significant flaws of many research studies, which tests for the toxicity of different chemicals is that they frequently will check these chemicals individually and miss the effects caused when combining with other active and inactive ingredients, (Natural Endocrine Solutions, 2018).

Media tells us a lot about the effects of glyphosate sprayed on GMO crops, but very little is said about the impact of the other active ingredient used in Roundup, which is Dicamba. Both glyphosate and dicamba affect the hormones responsible for growth and development. Plants sprayed with these two chemicals (Roundup) experience abnormal growth that results in death. Signs that a pet or wild animal may have been exposed to dicamba include shortness of breath, muscle spasms, and the animal may produce a lot of salivae. Birds may also be exposed to dicamba by eating dicamba granules, and signs include wing drop, a loss of controlled movements, and weakness (NPIC, 2012).

If you are eating any type of processed or refined foods then there is an excellent chance that you are being exposed to the negative health consequences of glyphosate and dicamba, (Natural Endocrine Solutions, 2018):

> **Neurotoxicity and oxidative stress:** Damages nerve cells (Cattani, 2014), Roundup over stimulates the production of the neurotransmitter glutamate, which in turn can cause damage to the neurons. Also, the inhalation of glyphosate can cause DNA damage (Koller VJ, 2012).

> **Cardiovascular health:** This can have a negative effect on cardiovascular health, leading to direct cardiac electrophysiological changes, conduction blocks, and arrhythmias (Gress, 2015).

➢ **Breast cancer:** There is evidence that low and environmentally relevant concentrations of glyphosate possess estrogenic activity and can induce the growth of human breast cancer cells. This, of course, doesn't mean that glyphosate will cause breast cancer in most individuals exposed to it, but it might increase the risk in susceptible individuals. As a result, while everyone should try to minimize their exposure to GMOs, those with a family history of breast cancer might want to make a greater effort to avoid these foods, ((Thongprakaisang, 2013); see section on Product Look-Up codes to learn how to avoid fresh produce that may have these residues.

➢ **Liver detoxification:** Can inhibit liver enzymes needed for detoxification. These enzymes play an essential role in the production of bile acids and cholesterol, whereas dicamba and glyphosate can impair our body's ability to produce and use bile acids and cholesterol, all of which can lead to problems with our gallbladder, (Lorbek, 2011). There is also evidence that disrupting the production of bile acid can also promote the toxic accumulation of the mineral manganese in the brainstem, which can cause or be a contributing factor to conditions such as Parkinson's disease (Samsel, 2015).

➢ **Mineral deficiencies:** Dicamba and glyphosate are chelating agents. Physiologically they affect pH levels, copper, and zinc can be relatively strongly complexed with glyphosate, whereas iron, calcium, magnesium, and manganese are complexed to lesser degrees (Duke, 2012).

➢ **Microbiota changes:** The study showed that highly pathogenic bacteria such as Salmonella and Clostridium are highly resistant to glyphosate, while most of the beneficial bacteria were found to be moderate to highly susceptible. Another study showed that glyphosate had an inhibitory effect on some of the good bacteria in the gut, but increased the population of pathogenic species (Ackermann, 2015). In other words, dicamba and glyphosate can kill the good bacteria, while not harming the bad ones that cause diseases.

Some farmers who use Roundup technology, spray their fields first to kill off all other plant life, then they plant their Roundup Ready seeds. They respray Roundup throughout the growing season. And again, when their crops are fully grown, they can spray a more massive dose of Roundup that kills off all the plant life, including their Roundup-ready crops in the field, making harvesting their crop easier. The downside to this is that organic seeds cannot be planted in that soil until the Roundup is completely gone, because Roundup kills all forms of natural plant life. Also, crops sprayed with Roundup can retain its residue and be passed on to the consumer.

Many studies link this herbicide and Gurt technologies to such conditions as medication resistance, leaky-gut syndrome, learning disabilities, cancer, degenerative & neurological diseases, and infertility.

"Our studies show that glyphosate acts as a disruptor of mammalian activity from concentrations 100 times lower than the recommended use in agriculture; this is noticeable on human placental cells after only 18 hours, and it can also affect aromatase gene expression. It also partially disrupts the ubiquitous reductase activity but at higher concentrations. Its effects are allowed and amplified by at least 0.02% of the adjuvants present in Roundup, known to facilitate cell penetration, and this should be carefully considered in pesticide evaluation. The dilution of glyphosate in Roundup formulation may multiply its endocrine effect. Roundup may be thus considered as a potential endocrine disruptor. Moreover, at higher doses still below the classical agricultural dilutions, its toxicity on placental cells could induce some reproduction problems" (Richard, 2005).

The amount of residue left on crops that are sprayed prior to harvesting may vary. Multiple autoimmune and antibiotic resistance are linked to seeds containing its antidote (ISF, 2003).

Farmers in America used to save seeds from their best crops to grow the next year, but since the mid-1990's more than 70% of American farmland has been converted to support only GMO crops. These farmers must buy Roundup-ready seeds and Roundup each year.

Many countries have banned GURT seeds because their farmers do not want to buy these pricy seeds and pesticides. Multiple countries that allow GMO crops from the USA require the grains to be milled (crushed) prior to entry into their country so that aberrant seeds or residue on crops cannot inadvertently contaminate their organic environment.

Major concerns include cross-pollination that may destroy wildlife and organic farmer's crops. Another matter is the effect this DNA may have on the health of their consumers. Research in other countries has linked these crops to infertility, birth defects learning disabilities, memory problems in addition to the usual chronic conditions of diabetes, cancer, and heart disease. No other nation spends even half of what Americans do on medical care annually.

Biocides: Pesticides, Herbicides, Fungicides and Rodenticides

Biocides are any product used to control pests. They are widely used to prevent insects, rodents, weeds, bacteria, mold, and fungus from ruining crops. Pesticides can be either selective, in which they only target specific organic life or non-selective / broad-spectrum, which targets most pests. They are designed to repel or kill pests by disrupting their ability to internally manufacture enzymes, hormones, or neurotransmitters from the nutrients they consume. This causes malnutrition in many pests because they are unable to digest food, but pesticides can also cause neurological problems that affect the behavior of the pest.

> The federal Environmental Protection Agency (EPA), the Food and Drug Administration (FDA) and the US Department of Agriculture (USDA) all The EPA is responsible for regulating pesticides by enforcing the 1996 Food Quality Protection Act. The EPA registers pesticides for use in the USA, evaluates potential new pesticides and their proposed uses, reviews the safety of older pesticides, registers pesticide producers, and enforces pesticide requirements. EPA has enacted stricter safety standards for infants and children and restricted many OP pesticides from residential use in order to reduce exposures in children. The FDA oversees the safety of the U.S. food supply, which includes monitoring pesticide residues in food. The USDA National Organic Program sets labeling standards for raw, fresh, and processed products that contain organic agricultural ingredients. The USDA Pesticide Data Program collects, analyzes, and reports pesticide residues on agricultural products in the U.S. food supply, particularly those highly consumed by infants and children, (Ecogenetics, 2013).

Pesticides are developed through stringent regulation processes to assure their effectiveness with minimal impact on human health and the environment. Even so, risk assessments of pesticide use are not easy, nor are they a particularly accurate process. Many factors can affect the results of a risk analysis, which are used by the FDA, EPA, and USDA to determine safety. Toxicity levels depend on the type of pesticide used, the amount and timing of application, and environmental characteristics that can all vary the effectiveness of the pesticide as well as its retention in the crops. Other factors are the adsorption on soil colloids, the weather conditions prevailing after application, and how long the pesticide persists in the environment, (Damalas, 2011). One of the biggest concerns is whether those pesticides know the difference between pests and humans (EPA, 2018) (EPA, 2017) (Gross, 2019) (Owens, 2010).

TABLE 1 Categories of Pesticides and Major Classes

Pesticide category	Major Classes	Examples
Insecticides	Organophosphates	Malathion, methyl parathion, acephate
	Carbamates	Aldicarb, carbaryl, methomyl, propoxur
	Pyrethroids/pyrethrins	Cypermethrin, fenvalerate, permethrin
	Organochlorines	Lindane
	Neonicotinoids	Imidacloprid
	N-phenylpyrazoles	Fipronil
Herbicides	Phosphonates	Glyphosate
	Chlorophenoxy herbicides	2,4-D, mecoprop
	Dipyridyl herbicides	Diquat, paraquat
	Nonselective	Sodium chlorate
Rodenticides	Anticoagulants	Warfarin, brodifacoum
	Convulsants	Strychnine
	Metabolic poison	Sodium fluoroacetate
	Inorganic compounds	Aluminum phosphide
Fungicides	Thiocarbamates	Metam-sodium
	Triazoles	Fluconazole, myclobutanil, triadimefon
	Strobilurins	Pyraclostrobin, picoxystrobin
Fumigants	Halogenated organic	Methyl bromide, Chloropicrin
	Organic	Carbon disulfide, Hydrogen cyanide, Naphthalene
	Inorganic	Phosphine
Miscellaneous	Arsenicals	Lead arsenate, chromated copper arsenate, arsenic trioxide
	Pyridine	4-aminopyridine

(Council of Pediatric Health, 2012)

Environmental risks associated with pesticide-exposures are residues and byproducts in food, air, and water. Hazards can range from short-term such as skin and eye irritation, headaches, dizziness, and nausea or chronic conditions such as neurological and neuromuscular diseases, cancer, asthma, and diabetes. Biocide risks are difficult to clarify due to the involvement of various factors: Period and level of exposure, type of pesticide toxicity and persistence, and the environmental characteristics of the affected areas. Also, most symptoms or diseases caused by exposure to biocides are multi-causal (Kim, 2017). This means that not all people and animals react the same to exposures.

By the very nature of pesticides, which induces starvation by disrupting digestive enzymes and hormones of the pests, when residue remains on or is saturated into produce, it can also harm our natural gut flora or interfere with our production of hormones and enzymes. Children and the elderly are at higher risk of health problems. Vitamin deficiencies, as well as hormone and enzyme imbalances, can produce many health problems.

Bacillus thuringiensis (Bt) is one type of pesticide that has been considered organic and therefore used by farmers for decades. It is widely used on corn and cotton. It naturally produces proteins that are poisonous and kills many insects by making their stomach burst. More recently, researchers have realized Bt and its byproduct can harm the digestive system of humans by attacking healthy gut flora and burning holes in the intestines. This can cause problems such as leaky gut syndrome. It can remain in the body for long periods of time that eventually attacks the lungs and even eyes of those who consumed it (Group, 2013).

Another example is apples saturated with pesticides. These pesticides can pass through the digestive system into our large intestines, where the majority of our microbiota uses insoluble fiber. When these pesticides kill off our natural disease-fighting gut bacteria, it makes way for harmful microorganisms to take-over and breed disease processes, including the growth of cancerous tumors. Sending your child to school with an apple or any fruit that is saturated in pesticides may be causing poor health, hyperactivity, allergies, and a host of other chronic ailments.

"This statement presents the position of the American Academy of Pediatrics on pesticides. Pesticides are a collective term for chemicals intended to kill unwanted insects, plants, molds, and rodents. Children encounter pesticides daily and have unique susceptibilities to their potential toxicity. Acute poisoning risks are clear, and understanding of chronic health implications from both acute and chronic exposure are emerging. Epidemiologic evidence demonstrates associations between early-life exposure to pesticides and pediatric cancers, decreased cognitive function, and behavioral problems. Related animal toxicology studies provide supportive biological plausibility for these findings. Recognizing and reducing problematic exposures will require attention to current inadequacies in medical training, public health tracking, and regulatory action on pesticides. Ongoing research describing toxicologic vulnerabilities and exposure factors across the life span are needed to inform regulatory needs and appropriate interventions. Policies that promote integrated pest management, comprehensive pesticide labeling, and marketing practices that incorporate child health considerations will enhance safe use (Council of Pediatric Health, 2012).

"In accordance with the 1990 Farm Bill, all Private Applicators of Pesticides were required by law to keep a record(s) of their federally restricted use pesticide (RUP) applications for a period of 2 years. These operations ended in September 2013 due to the elimination of program funding by our legislators" (USDA, 2016). Recent studies determined that 70% of conventionally grown produce has pesticide residue on its skin.

When pesticides are sprayed on natural plant life, rainwater flushes them into streams and lakes, and then those chemicals wreak havoc with the earth's natural purification system. Anything that harms the environment will also harm humans and other animals when exposed to it in any way.

"The Pesticide Data Program (PDP) is a national pesticide residue monitoring program and produces the most comprehensive pesticide residue database in the U.S. The Monitoring Programs Division administers PDP activities, including the sampling, testing, and reporting of pesticide residues on agricultural commodities in the U.S. food supply, with an emphasis on those commodities highly consumed by infants and children. The program is implemented through cooperation with State agriculture departments and other Federal agencies. PDP data:

- Enable the U.S. Environmental Protection Agency to assess dietary exposure.

- Facilitate the global marketing of U.S. agricultural products.

- Provide guidance for the U.S. Food and Drug Administration and other governmental agencies to make informed decisions" (USDA, 2019) (Schepker, 2018).

It is important to note that just because a pesticide residue is detected on a fruit or vegetable, it does not mean it is unsafe. Tiny amounts of pesticides that may remain in or on fruits, vegetables, grains, and other foods decrease as crops are harvested, transported, exposed to light, washed, prepared, and cooked. The presence of a detectable pesticide residue does not mean the residue is at an unsafe level. USDA's Pesticide Data Program (PDP) detects residues at levels far lower than those that are considered health risks.

The best way to avoid illness caused by pesticide residue or byproducts is to buy organic. When purchasing products that may have chemical residue on the skin, wash thoroughly, and remove the skin. If you use the zest of oranges or lemons peels in cooking, the best way to assure you are not putting any harmful chemicals into your baked goods is to buy organic.

If you are concerned about pesticide ingestion, there are home test kits that detect pesticide residue, which is similar to pregnancy dipstick tests, only more complex (Schepker, 2018) (Abraxis, 2017).

Three primary warnings regarding pesticide effects on human health and our environment are (Council of Pediatric Health, 2012):

1. Consumer awareness: Pesticide exposures are common and cause both acute and chronic effects. Exposure includes residues on food, household products and community, workplace, and school use of pesticide products.
2. Medical providers need to be more aware of and be knowledgeable in pesticide identification, counseling, and management
3. Governmental actions to improve pesticide safety are needed. Whenever a new public policy is developed, or existing policy is revised, the full range of consequences of pesticide use on children and their families should be considered.

Fortified with Food Additives, Preservatives, and Chemicals

Food additives have been used by people for centuries to improve the quality of what is consumed. "Our ancestors used salt to preserve meats and fish, added herbs and spices to improve the flavor of foods, preserved fruit with sugar, and pickled cucumbers in a vinegar solution," (FDA, 2010). While many of these methods are still being used, in more recent decades, many synthetic chemicals and food additives made from GMOs have been approved and added to processed foods. Their intended purposes include: Increase nutrient value, enhance flavor, improve odor and visual appearance, improve texture and stability, and/or prevent spoilage.

When the FDA determines an additive is Generally Recognized as Safe (GRAS), this is not a guarantee that the additive is always safe. It merely means there are fewer circumstances when they have harmful effects than safe effects when consumed. In many cases, food additives and chemicals are safe when consumed in a single serving size each day and not every day.

The problem with this is that the food industry has been allowed to use various names for the same food additives. Thereby, consumers may not realize they are consuming toxic levels of chemicals and food additives that may have immediate consequences or evolve over a long period of time when they consume different foods that contain the same additive only under a different name.

When common organic ingredients are added to processed foods, they are reliably listed as what they are commonly known as, such as nutmeg is always called nutmeg, and water is always called water. But often different food manufactures that put POB-foods-additives and chemicals into their meals use many different names on their ingredient panel for the same additive. For instance, high fructose corn syrup may also be referred to as HFCS, Corn syrup, maize syrup, tapioca syrup, glucose/fructose syrup, glucose syrup, dahlia syrup, and crystalline glucose, all of which are digested into the same compound, (Hunt, n.d.).

By using different names for the same additive, the food industry is able to fool and confuse the consumer. Ingredients on food labels are listed in the order of the highest amount to the least amount of each food ingredient (FDA, 2010). For instance, if high fructose us the second most abundant ingredient used in a food product, it should be listed as the second ingredient, but some unscrupulous food manufacturers may list it as the fifth ingredient -high fructose corn syrup, the sixth ingredient corn syrup, the seventh ingredient maize, and the tenth ingredient glucose syrup. Fundamentally, when you add all of the amounts up, they are the same ingredient, which is the second-largest amount of food in that product.

Food companies take advantage of the name change to hide ingredients they feel the public may want to avoid if made aware.

Legally, the food additive term refers to any substance intended to directly or indirectly affect the characteristics of a food-product (FDA, 2010):

☺ Direct food additives: Ingredients added to a food for a specific purpose in that food. For example, xanthan gum used in salad dressings, chocolate milk, bakery fillings, puddings, and other foods to add texture. Most direct additives are identified on the ingredient label of foods

☺ Indirect food additives: Ingredients that become part of the food in trace amounts due to its packaging, storage, or other handling. For instance, minute amounts of packaging substances may find their way into foods during storage. Food packaging manufacturers must prove to the U.S. Food and Drug Administration (FDA) that all materials coming in contact with food are safe before they are permitted for use in such a manner

Extensive scientific evidence is available that proves the negative health consequences of many food additives that can affect some of the people all of the time and a lot of people some of the time when consumed in more portions than one serving daily or consumed in large amounts over long periods of time. The bottom line is, food additives are used to control mother nature of which humans are part of. Many food additives have benefits that outweigh the risks, and for those who are not at risk, the benefits are better preservation of those foods. Therefore, the best way to protect yourself is to become informed about food additives and avoid processed foods that contain ingredients that cause your specific symptoms.

The FDA maintains a list of over 3000 ingredients in its database named "Everything Added to Food in the United States" (FDA, 2019).

Types of food additives include (FDA, 2010):

☺ **Preservatives: Used to maintain or improve safety and freshness.** Preservatives slow product spoilage caused by mold, air, bacteria, fungi, or yeast. In addition to maintaining the quality of the food, they help control contamination that can cause foodborne illness, including life-threatening botulism. One group of preservatives known as antioxidants prevents fats and oils and the foods containing them from becoming rancid or developing an off-flavor. They also prevent cut fresh fruits such as apples from turning brown when exposed to air

☺ **Fortified Additives: Increase or help maintain Nutritional Value.** Vitamins and minerals (and fiber) are added to many foods to make up for those lacking in a person's diet or lost in processing or to enhance the nutritional quality of a consumable-product. Such fortification and enrichment have helped reduce malnutrition in the U.S. and worldwide. All products containing added nutrients must be appropriately labeled

☺ **Spices, Natural and Artificial Flavors, and Sweeteners**: Are added to enhance the taste of food. Food colors maintain or improve their appearance

☺ **Color Additives:** Are used to enhance the appeal of foods

☺ **Emulsifiers, Stabilizers, and Thickeners:** Give foods the texture and consistency consumers expect

☺ **Leavening Agents:** Allow baked goods to rise during baking

Not all FDA approved food additives are approved in other countries, so if you are experiencing any health problems, mental or physical, look up the additives in the foods you regularly consume to see if your symptoms may be caused by those additives. If you are healthy with no indications of illness, probably the food additives you consume are in portions that cannot harm you, and therefore their benefits outweigh their risks.

Cloned, Trans-genetic & Test-tube Meats

"Lab-grown meat would free up producers from being dependent on farms by allowing for real beef to be made in a lab from animal cells instead of from slaughter. New technologies like CRISPR allow us to safely increase the quality of our cell growth, which means we will make meat that is tastier, healthier, and more sustainable, according to the founder and CEO of a current clone-meat manufacturer" (Brodwin, 2019).

America is about three decades into the GMO food technology movement, and finally, scientists have created lab-made meats that can be sold for as little as $2000 a pound of ground beef or $250 per hamburger, whereas a link of sausage is about $2500. Both are requiring blood genes from multiple pregnant cows to supply the blood. "Impossible Foods CEO Patrick Brown says his goal is to one day replace the meat industry altogether" (Purdy, 2017). In the meantime, it is being subsidized by Now, all we need is an Affordable Food Act, so our taxes can be used to make these affordable to everyone.

Impossible Burger received $75 million in subsidized investments from Singapore-based venture fund Temasek, Bill Gates, Khosla Ventures, and others. These supporters helped bring this company's total funding to over $250 million to bring the cost down low enough for average consumers to buy (Robinson M. , 2017). Keep in mind that many people do not buy organic food because it is too expensive in supermarkets. They sacrifice the quality and safety over cost. Why can't this amount of money be invested in organic food to make it more affordable?

Currently, less than one-third of all cloned and trans-genetic animals turn out as intended. The other two-thirds are destroyed and disposed of in a manner that is not intended to pose a threat to the natural environment. These genetically altered animals require thousands of acres of farmland to house and feed.

Functional Foods

Functional food is a cute way of implying that foods with medical implications are healthy and safe to consume. When consumed in recommended amounts as indicated on labels as a serving size, most additives are safe for anyone who does not have any illnesses. But those additives can add up when more substantial portions or many foods containing those additives are consumed. We can unknowingly be over-dosing ourselves. When we eat an entire package that may include many servings, those health-intended additives may be crossing over into the over-dosing gray area. Remember that our liver and kidneys must filter toxins and food. Many Americans are eating foods that contain medications, residues, and chemicals that alter their growth, immunity, and fertility, as well as a host of other health problems, (Whitman, 2014). When the FDA deems a food additive to be Generally Recognized as Safe (GRAS), they base their opinion on the amount in a single serving. How many people eat only ten potato chips or an ounce of candy throughout a day and then no other foods with those additives for at least 24 hours?

The more processed foods consumed, the higher the likeliness that you are consuming toxic levels of chemicals that may take years to impair you fully. In the meantime, consumers adapt to the mild symptoms caused by these processed foods.

Conclusion

POB food changes the composition of organic food; therefore, their products do not contain the same nutrients. When preparing a meal, if you substitute ingredients, the finished product will not be the same. For example, if you substitute chocolate with strawberries when baking a cake, the end product will not taste like chocolate, it will have a different number of calories, and it is merely not a chocolate cake. So, when the food industry tells us milk from cows that have human genes produce the same quality of milk, they are not telling the truth. Why would these companies spend so much time and money on altering genes if they generate the same product as nature?

The US Elected officials over the past 25 years have passed laws that allow the POB food industry to conceal ingredients that may cause health problems. When Americans unite to start demanding elected officials sign the Cartagena Act and make labeling of all foods accurate and transparent, we will be empowered to make better-informed healthy choices about the foods we consume.

POB foods are intended to control Mother Nature; unregulated biotechnology not only causes many illnesses, but it also causes a shortage of organic food supplies. The money and organic life used to support POB research could be used to help farmers, increase job security, and grow healthy foods that are naturally affordable.

Key Points

♣ There are at least ninety nutrients needed throughout life to maintain vitality and continuously restore worn-out cells and tissues

♣ Generally Recognized as Safe is a term used by the FDA to indicate that most people, but not all, will probably not experience any harmful effects by consuming GRAS food additives

♣ The ideal treatment for illnesses caused by consumption of toxic additives and pesticide residues is to stop eating food that contains those ingredients

♣ The difference between organic and genetically engineered foods is how crops and animals come to life.

♣ Organic food is the opposite of POB processed foods

♣ When scientists change the genes of a plant or animals, the new product will contain different nutrients

♣ Scientific studies appraise the effects of toxins individually. The outcomes of individual toxins, when combined with other ingredients or toxins, are often unknown until products containing these combinations are already being sold to Americans.

♣ Many processed and GMO foods are subsidized with millions of dollars to bring down their costs so that average consumers can afford to buy them. Organic food is not subsidized, and therefore consumers are tricked into thinking processed, and GMO foods are cheaper to manufacture than organic food.

♣ When you buy unhealthy processed foods, you are supporting that industry. When you stop buying unhealth processed foods, that is the most effective way to get it removed from our supermarket shelves.

REFERENCES

Ackermann, W. C. (2015). The influence of glyphosate on the microbiota and production of botulinum neurotoxin during ruminal fermentation. *Current Microbiology*, 374-382.

Acousta, L. (2014). *Restrictions on Genetically Modified Organisms.* Retrieved from The Law Library of Congress, Global Legal Research Center, p. 208 -212: http://www.loc.gov/law/help/restrictions-on-gmos/restrictions-on-gmos.pdf

AFCC. (2017). *General infertility: Causes, testing, and treatment.* Retrieved from Advanced Fertility Center in Chicago: https://www.advancedfertility.com/infertility.htm

Amedeo, K. (2018). *The rising cost of healthcare by year and its causes.* Retrieved from The Balance : https://www.thebalance.com/causes-of-rising-healthcare-costs-4064878

Bethell, C. K. (2011). A national and state profile of leading health problems and health care quality for US children: key insurance disparities and across-state variations. *Academy of Pediatric Medicine*, S22-33.

Better gardening. (2019). *Cow manure fertilizer supercharging your garden.* Retrieved from Better Gardening : https://www.bettervegetablegardening.com/cow-manure-fertilizer.html

Bonn, D. (2005). Roundup Revelation: Weed Killer Adjuvants May Boost Toxicity. *Environmental Health Perspective, 113 (6)*, A403–A404.

Brodwin, E. (2019). *Silicon Valley startups backed by celebrities like Bill Gates are using gene-editing tool CRISPR to make meat without farms and to disrupt a $200 billion industry.* Retrieved from Business Insider: https://www.businessinsider.com/silicon-valley-startups-using-crispr-chicken-beef-memphis-meats-new-age-meats-2019-3

Cattani, D. L.-C.-C. (2014). *Mechanisms underlying the neurotoxicity induced by glyphosate-based herbicide in immature rat hippocampus: Involvement of glutamate excitotoxicity.* Retrieved from Toxicology, 320: 34-45

CDC. (2019). *Reproductive health: Teen pregnancy.* Retrieved from Center for Disease Prevention: https://www.cdc.gov/teenpregnancy/about/index.htm

Center for Food Safety. (2018). *AquaAdvantage salmon.* Retrieved from CenterforFoodSafty.org: https://www.centerforfoodsafety.org/issues/309/ge-fish/aquadvantage-salmon

Convention on Biodiversity. (1999). Consequences of the use of the new technology for the control of plant gene expression for the conservation and sustainable use of biological diversity. Montreal: UNEP/CBD/SBSTTA/4/9/Rev.1.

Cordain, L. B.-M. (2010). Origins and evolution of the Western diet: health implications for the 21st century. *The American Journal of Clinical Nutrition*, 331-354.

Council of Pediatric Health. (2012). *Policy Statement: Pesticide exposure in children.* Retrieved from Pediatrics 130 (6): Council on Environmental Health: www.pediatrics.org/cgi/doi/10.1542/peds.2012-2757

Devereux, G. (2006). The increase in the prevalence of asthma and allergy: food for thought. *Nat'l Review of Immunology, 11*, 869-874.

Drugs.com. (2018). *Organic Food: Are they Safer to Eat.* Retrieved from Drugs.com: https://www.drugs.com/mca/organic-foods-are-they-safer-more-nutritious

Dubock, A. (2014). The present status of golden rice. *Journal of Huazhong Agricultural University, No. 6 (v33)*, 69 - 84.

Duke, S. O. (2012). Glyphosate effects on plant mineral nutrition, crop rhizosphere microbiota, and plant disease in glyphosate-resistant crops. *Journal of Agriculture and Food Chemistry, 60(42)*, 10375-10397.

Ecogenetics. (2013). *Health Risks of Pesticides in Food.* University of Washington: The Center for Ecogenetics and Environment Health, University of Washington, 1/2013. NIEHS Grant #ESO7033. Retrieved from Center for Ecogenetics.

EHS. (2017). *Biohazard disposal.* Retrieved from University of Texas, Dept of Environmental Health & Safety (EHS): https://ehs.utexas.edu/programs/biosafety/biohazardous-waste-disposal.php

EPA. (2018). *Pesticide use in NSW.* Retrieved from Environmental Protective Agency: https://www.epa.nsw.gov.au/your-environment/pesticides/pesticide-use-nsw

Everding, G. (2016). *Genetically modified Golden Rice falls short on lifesaving promises.* Retrieved from the Source: Science & Technology: https://source.wustl.edu/2016/06/genetically-modified-golden-rice-falls-short-lifesaving-promises/

FDA. (2010). *Overview of food ingredients, additives, and color.* Retrieved from Food and Drug Administration: https://www.fda.gov/food/food-ingredients-packaging/overview-food-ingredients-additives-colors

FDA. (2019). *Everything added to food in the USA.* Retrieved from FDA: http://www.comfortncolor.com/HTML/Pittsfield%20paper/Everything%20A dded%20to%20Food%20in%20the%20United%20States%20(EAFUS).pdf

Flanders, W. (2018). *The Flavr Savr tomato.* Retrieved from Flanders health blog: https://www.flandershealth.us/genetic-engineering/the-flavr-savr-tomato.html

Foss, A. (2012). *Growing fatter on a GMO diet.* Retrieved from Science Nordic: http://sciencenordic.com/growing-fatter-gm-diet

Foster, K. (2016). *Toxic legacy: Monsanto and PCB contamination.* Retrieved from Waterkeeper: https://waterkeeper.org/toxic-legacy-monsanto-and-pcb-contamination/

Genetic Literacy Program. (2016). *Which genetically engineered crops and animals are approved in the US?* Retrieved from Genetic Literacy Program: https://gmo.geneticliteracyproject.org/FAQ/which-genetically-engineered-crops-are-approved-in-the-us/

GMO FAQ. (2018). *Where are GMO crops and animals approved and banned?* https://gmo.geneticliteracyproject.org/FAQ/where-are-gmos-grown-and-banned/: Science Literacy Program.

GMO Science. (2015). *Are GMOs contributing to the rise in chronic health conditions in our children?* Retrieved from GMO Science: https://www.gmoscience.org/777-2/

GMO Science. (2015). *Top five childhood diseases on the rise.* Retrieved from GMO Science: https://www.gmoscience.org/top-five-childhood-diseases-rise/

Gold, M. (2007, 2018). *Organic production/ organic food: Information access tools.* Retrieved from United States Department of Agriculture: https://www.nal.usda.gov/afsic/organic-productionorganic-food-information-access-tools#systems

Goodman, B. (2015). *Anything fishy about genetically altered fish?* Retrieved from WebMD: https://www.webmd.com/food-recipes/news/20151119/genetically-modified-salmon-fda#1

Greger, M. (2012). The welfare of transgenetic farm animals. In P. R. Sammour, *Biotechnology- Molecular Studies and Novel Applications for Improved Quality of Human Life* (pp. 46 - 64). Tanta, Egypt: Tanta University. Retrieved from www.intechopen.com / Humane Society of the USA.

Gress, S. L. (2015). Glyphosate-based herbicides potently affect the cardiovascular system in mammals: Review of the literature. *Cardiovascular Toxicology, 115(2)*, 117-126.

Haefs R, S.-E. M. (2002). Studies on a new group of biodegradable surfactants for glyphosate. *Pest management science, 58.*, 825-833.

Halfon, N. H. (2012). The changing landscape of disability in childhood. *The Future of Children 22(1):13-42,* 13-42.

Harmon, C. (2009). *Cracked corn: Scientists solve maize's corn maze.* Retrieved from Scientific American: https://www.scientificamerican.com/article/corn-genome-cracked/

Hauck, D. (2014). *Supreme Court hands Monsanto victory over farmers on GMO seed patents, ability to sue .* Retrieved from USA News; Reuters: https://www.rt.com/usa/monsanto-patents-sue-farmers-547/

Hayden, K. (2011). *Children of the Corn: GMO Sterility and Spermicides.* Retrieved from Truthistreason.net: http://www.truthistreason.net/children-of-the-corn-gmo-sterility-and-spermicides

Hertz-Picciotto, I. D. (2009). The rise in autism and the role of age at diagnosis. *Epidemiology, 20(1),* 84-90.

Highfructosecornsyrup.org. (2009). *Guess what's lurking in your food.* Retrieved from Highfructosecornsyrup.org: http://www.highfructosecornsyrup.org/2009/02/guess-whats-lurking-in-your-food.html

Hilbeck, A. e. (2015). *No scientific consensus that GMOs are safe.* Environmental Science, 27(4).

Hunt, T. (n.d.). *8 Fake names for high fructose corn syrup.* Retrieved from Dr. Tunis: http://drtunisjr.com/8-fake-names-for-high-fructose-corn-syrup/

Institute of Transformative Bio-Molecules . (2017). *Plant's parent genes cooperate in shaping their child: Discovery of parental factors that lead to asymmetric division of the zygote.* Retrieved from Science Daily: https://www.sciencedaily.com/releases/2017/04/170421103747.htm

ISF. (2003). *Genetic Use Restriction Technologies.* Retrieved from International Seed Federation: https://www.worldseed.org/wp-content/uploads/2015/10/Genetic_Use_Restriction_Technologies_20030611_En1.pdf

Koller VJ, F. M. (2012). Cytotoxic and DNA-damaging properties of glyphosate and Roundup in human-derived buccal epithelial cells. *Toxicology, 86(5),* 805-813.

Koon, R. (2007). *Carrageenan information issues and .* Retrieved from DietStandards.com: https://dietstandards.com/wp-content/uploads/Carrageenan-Information-Issues.pdf

Lapidus, F. (2018). *Studies estimate a shortage of insulin by 2030.* Retrieved from Science & Health Broadcast: https://www.voanews.com/a/study-estimates-shortage-of-insulin-by-2030/4671590.html

Lewis, A. (2017). *Why do some crops contain Epicyte?* Retrieved from Holistic, healthy living: https://www.holistichealthliving.com/why-do-some-gm-crops-contain-the-epicyte-gene/

Linabery, A. R. (2008). Trends in childhood cancer incidence in the U.S. (1992-2004). *Cancer, 112(2),* 416-432.

Lipman, T. L.-K. (2013). Increasing incidence of type 1 diabetes in youth: twenty years of the Philadelphia Pediatric Diabetes Registry. *Diabetes Care, 36(6),* 1597-1603.

Lorbek, G. L. (2011). Cytochrome P450s in the synthesis of cholesterol and bile acids – from mouse models to human diseases. *The FEBS Journal, 279(8),* 1516-1533.

Madden, J. (2013). *Carrageenan and celiac disease.* Retrieved from The patient celiac: http://www.thepatientceliac.com/2013/01/13/carrageenan-and-celiac-disease/

Mahdi, B. S. (2011). Frequency of anti-sperm antibodies in infertile women. *Journal of Reproductive Infertility, 12(4),* 261–265.

Main, E. (2012). *Are GMOs making you fat?* Rodale.

Majda, W. (2014). *Is feeding animals with manure the way to go?* Retrieved from Designer Ecosystems: http://designerecosystems.com/2014/07/12/is-feeding-animals-with-manure-the-way-to-go/

Malaty, H. F. (2010). Rising incidence of inflammatory bowel disease among children: a 12-year study. *Journal Pediatric Gastroenterol Nutrition, 50(1),* 27-31.

McComb, B. (2016). *GMO's can help combat world hunger.* Retrieved from The Borgen Project: https://borgenproject.org/gmos-world-hunger/

McKie, R. (2001). GMO Corn Set to Stop Man Spreading His Seed. *The Observer, London.*

Minako Ueda, M. A. (2017). Transcriptional integration of paternal and maternal factors in the Arabidopsis zygote. *Genes & Development, 31 (6),* 617.

Moss, L. (2010). *Banana vaccines.* Retrieved from Mother Nature : https://www.mnn.com/green-tech/research-innovations/photos/12-bizarre-examples-of-genetic-engineering/banana-vaccines#top-desktop

Natural Endocrine Solutions. (2018). *Does glyphosate have a negative effect on thyroid health?* Retrieved from Natural Endocrine Solutions: https://www.naturalendocrinesolutions.com/articles/does-glyphosate-have-a-negative-effect-on-thyroid-health/

NIHCD. (2012). *Focus on Infertility Research at the NICHD.* Retrieved from National Institute of Health Child Health and Human Development: https://www.nichd.nih.gov/newsroom/resources/spotlight/061512-infertility

Nolte, K. (n.d.). *Soy Beans.* Retrieved from Yuma County Extention; Arizona Edu: https://cals.arizona.edu/fps/sites/cals.arizona.edu.fps/files/cotw/Soybeans.pdf

NPIC. (2012). *Dicamba general fact sheet.* Retrieved from National Pesticide Information Center: http://npic.orst.edu/factsheets/dicamba_gen.html

Olsen, R. S. (2016). *In a new survey of eleven countries, US adults still struggle with access to and affordability of health care.* Retrieved from Health Affairs: https://www.healthaffairs.org/doi/abs/10.1377/hlthaff.2016.1088

Onusic, S. (2013). *Violent Behavior: A solution in plain sight.* Retrieved from The Weston A. Price Foundation: https://www.westonaprice.org/health-topics/environmental-toxins/violent-behavior-a-solution-in-plain-sight/

Owens, K. F. (2010). *Wide range of diseases linked to pesticides.* Retrieved from Pesticides and You, 30 (2) pages 13 - 21: https://www.beyondpesticides.org/assets/media/documents/health/pid-database.pdf

Radhakrishnan, D. D. (2014). Trends in the age of diagnosis of childhood asthma. *J Allergy Clin Immunol. 134(5),* S1057 - 1062.

Richard, S. M. (2005). Differential effects of glyphosate and roundup on human placental cells and aromatase. *Environmental Health Perspectives, 113(6),* 716 - 720.

Samsel, A. S. (2015). Glyphosate, pathways to modern diseases III: Manganese, neurological diseases, and associated pathologies. *Surgical Neurology International, 6(45).*

SARE. (ND). *The history of organic farming in the United States.* Retrieved from Sustainable Agriculture Research & Education: https://www.sare.org/Learning-Center/Bulletins/Transitioning-to-Organic-Production/Text-Version/History-of-Organic-Farming-in-the-United-States

Segedie, L. (2019). *There's WHAT in My Sandwich? Detoxing Unhealthy Peanut Butter.* Retrieved from Mamavation: https://www.mamavation.com/featured/detoxing-unhealthy-peanut-butters.html

Shapiro, A. M. (2008). Fructose-induced leptin resistance exacerbates weight gain in response to subsequent high-fat feeding. *American Journal of J Physiol Regul Integr Comp Physiol., 295 (5)*, R1370–R1375.

Shiva, V. (2018). *Seeds of suicide: Hoe Monsanto destroys farming.* Retrieved from Global Research: https://www.globalresearch.ca/the-seeds-of-suicide-how-monsanto-destroys-farming/5329947

Simmons, A. J. (2015). What are we putting in the food that Is making us fat? Food additives, contaminants, and other putative contributors to obesity. *Curr Obes Rep., 3(2)*, 273-285.

Swanson, N. (2013). *Mounting evidence that GMO crops can cause infertility and birth defects.* Seattle Examiner.

The Cornucopia Institute. (2016). *Carrageenan: New studies reinforce the link to inflammation, cancer, and diabetes.* Retrieved from The Cornucopia Institute: https://www.cornucopia.org/wp-content/uploads/2016/04/CarageenanReport-2016.pdf

The Guardian News. (2019). *GM corn set to stop the spread of man's seed.* Retrieved from The Guardian New: https://www.theguardian.com/science/2001/sep/09/gm.food

Thongprakaisang, S. T. (2013). Glyphosate induces human breast cancer cells growth via estrogen receptors. *Food Chemistry Toxicology*, 129-136.

Tonti-Filippini, N. (2001). *Ethics and human-animal transgenesis.* 1 - 13: L'Osservatore Romano supplement article .

USDA. (nd). *Organic Foods Protection Act .* Retrieved from United States Department of Agriculture: national standard for organic food and fiber production

Walia, A. (2014). *10 scientific studies are proving GMOs can be harmful to human health.* Retrieved from Awareness: https://www.collective-evolution.com/2014/04/08/10-scientific-studies-proving-gmos-can-be-harmful-to-human-health/

Waminal, O. R. (2013). Randomly Detected Genetically Modified (GM) Maize (Zea mays L.) near a Transport Route Revealed a Fragile 45S rDNA Phenotype. *PLoS One, 8(9)*, e74060. .

Weiner, S. (2018). *American life expectancy will rank 64th globally by 2040, new data shows.* Retrieved from Healthcare: https://splinternews.com/americans-will-rank-64th-in-global-life-expectancy-by-2-1829923357

Wong, A. C. (2016). Genetically modified foods in China and the United States: A primer of regulation and intellectual property protection. *Food Science and Human Wellness, 5(3)*, 124 - 140.

Woodson, W. (2004). *Transgenic and cloned food animal guidelines for Purdue University*. Lafayette, IN: Purdue University.

Yu, C. (2018). *Is the impossible burger really better for you than a regular burger?* Retrieved from Women's Health: https://www.womenshealthmag.com/food/a21050196/the-impossible-burger/

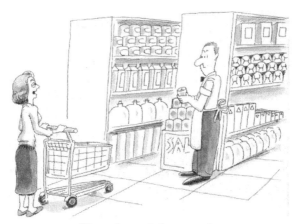

"In what aisle are the
'won't immediately kill you' foods?"

Chapter 8
Food Laws and Labels

Most Americans, including myself, want to make good food choices. Therefore, the more we know about American food laws and labels, the easier it is to select foods that keep us healthy while avoiding those that harm us immediately or over many years. Understanding labeling laws are crucial for all consumers. Do you know what labels are and are not telling you?

Most consumers assume all foods sold in supermarkets are safe. We trust that our federally funded government agencies ban any foods that can harm any of us and that all new genetically engineered foods are thoroughly tested for safety before selling to the public. But this is not always true. Foods that are Generally Recognized as Safe (GRAS) by our FDA are not guaranteed to be safe for consumption because they are not regulated by the FDA or USDA. As stated in chapter 7, food that comes from plants or animals is not necessarily what they are labeled unless they are certified organic. GMO food producers are self-regulated.

Comparing America food laws with countries that signed the Cartagena Act, those other countries require food products to be proven safe prior to its sale, whereas in the USA, GRAS food is assumed safe until proven otherwise. For example, American consumers are currently experiencing an influx of plant-based hamburgers that look and smell like beef with a special sauce that resembles blood to imitate like real meat. These burgers are made from GMO soy and are high in saturated fat. It is arguably intended to replace beef and, eventually, other meat products, but its effects on human health are unknown and yet to be determined. As gluten is the protein in some grains, the impossible burger is using soy and yeast protein.

> "While it's unlikely that these yeast proteins are overtly toxic, the yeast does not seem to have been part of the human diet, so we don't know if it could cause immune reactions and allergies. Impossible Foods argued against allergenicity, partly on the basis that a bioinformatics analysis using the Allergenonline database did not show a greater than 35% similarity to known allergenic proteins" (GMO Science, 2018).

Many derivatives from GMO soy are in most processed food in the American supermarket. The food industry has replaced much of the American diet with imitation food made from GMO soy: Soymilk, soy butter, soy cheese, soy meat, soy oil in peanut butter, and salad dressing. A well-balanced diet cannot depend on one plant, and doing so will inevitably cause malnutrition because every human requires at least ninety different nutrients that come from a variety of natural plants and animals. A healthy diet consists of a variety of plant and animal foods. Ultimately this is contributing to the increase in chronic illness and increase demand for medical care.

If the unregulated GMO food industry is eliminating its organic competition, all Americans should be examining which politicians (our public servants) are being made rich by this industry, because future laws about farming, organic food and the safety of food ingredients sold in supermarkets will be heavily influenced those we elect to represent our interest.

> "Why the Impossible Burger cannot be stopped: The beef industry has started to quiver, and rightfully so: Word comes out today that, flush with untold capital, Impossible Foods has apparently decided to spend some of it on a Washington lobbyist. Back in 2016, the Good Food Institute formed with backing from people at Memphis Meats, Just (formerly Hampton Creek), and other "clean meat" start-ups. Today, it's got a lobbying arm that

represents the industry's interests, but Washington *Post* tech reporter Tony Romm tweeted this morning that Impossible Foods filed the necessary paperwork back on February 20 to hire its own dedicated team — suggesting it plans to start bringing the heat to win over elected officials to the high-tech meat-substitute cause, (Rainer, 2018).

As GMO foods increasingly replaced organic food over the past decade, Americans are deliberately misled into thinking these unlabeled novelty foods are healthy, all the while the cost of medical care to treat its chronic effects have become unaffordable. When new under-tested and unregulated genetically engineered foods are released into the marketplace, their adverse effects are yet to be discovered, and most often, medical professionals do not connect the release of new GMO food with the development of a new disease or chronic illness. Most medical professionals are unaware of the side-effects of GMO foods and, therefore, can only treat the symptoms while their patients continue to consume the GMO foods, chemicals, and additives that are causing their illnesses.

American consumers simply depend on elected representatives to make laws that protect us while the food industry lobbies those same legislators.

"In 2012 alone, companies spent over $30 million "influencing" Congress on agricultural issues, including making sure they didn't pass legislation that would label GMOs or outlaw them altogether. Is it any wonder that the United States of America is one of the very last nations in the world to either ban GMOs outright or require their labeling on foods?" (Adams, 2013)

"OpenSecrets.org, a project of the Center for Responsive Politics, reported that, as of July 21, Monsanto had already spent over $2.5 million dollars on lobbying this year. The corporation is on track to meet or beat last year's 2014 spending total, which reached $4,120,000. Yet it doesn't appear to be on pace to break the record the company set for itself in 2008 when it spent $9 million on lobbying.

At the federal level, Monsanto's millions are spent to ensure Congress passes laws that work in the company's favor. The corporation lobbied heavily for the Safe and Accurate Food Labeling Act of 2015, better known to food safety activists as the "DARK Act," which would overrule hundreds of local laws regulating the labeling of foods containing genetically-modified ingredients with a still undeveloped USDA program," (O'Connel, 2015)

In 1989, a lot of research warned of the harmful effects of aspartame, but lobbyists influenced legislators who then approved its use in low-calorie products. Since then, researchers have concluded aspartame causes many mental and physical illnesses, while our legislators continue to protect its producer's ability to be put into most diet drinks and other products (Starr-Hull, 2014). Now, in 2019, we have vegan-meat-that-bleeds imitation GMO soy blood. Its lobbyists are funding current legislation before its effects on healthcare are known (Rainer, 2018).

Legislators, congressmen, and presidents had played major roles in the safety and quality of food sold in America since as far back as 1862 when Abraham Lincoln created the United States Department of Agriculture (USDA). He had the foresight to understand the potential risks the industrial age posed and passed legislation to protect our farmland and the environment. Then came the federal consumer protection agency with the passage of the 1906 Pure Food and Drugs Act by Theodore Roosevelt; this is now our Food and Drug Administration (FDA). Around that same time, a book called *The Jungle* by Sinclair Upton made the public aware of the unsanitary meatpacking conditions, which led to the Meat Packers Act of that same year, 1906.

During the Great Depression, President Roosevelt passed into law the Farm Bill.

"The Farm Bill was originally created in 1933 as part of President Franklin D. Roosevelt's *Agricultural Adjustment Act,* which provided subsidies to U.S. farmers in the midst of the Great Depression. The federal government paid farmers to stop the production of seven main crops, known as "commodities," in the hopes of decreasing the supply and thus increasing the prices of staple crops. The Act also contained several provisions related to conservation, support for farmers suffering from effects of the Dust Bowl, and the storage of surplus harvests. the Act was later declared unconstitutional by the Supreme Court (the tax structure used to fund the program was deemed an overreach of the powers of the federal government), its basic premise was included in later *Agricultural Adjustment Acts* and eventually became the basis for all future U.S. Farm Bills. Since 1965, Farm Bills have been passed with general consistency every five or six years. The 2014 Farm Bill provided $489 billion in mandatory spending over the next five years. According to the Congressional Research Service, the 2014 Farm Bill restructures support for traditional commodity crops—grains, oilseeds, and cotton—by eliminating direct payments. Currently, most support for farmers comes from crop insurance programs in which farmers only receive payments when prices or revenues decrease." (Snap to Health, 2019).

Around 1958 the food labeling act was passed, which is still used today. Some consumer advocates blame misleading labeling by the food industry on this outdated piece legislation (Sixwise.com, 2009). Much of the cultivation and added ingredients remain voluntary information for the producers to decide whether or not to disclose specific information about their product.

Due to many reported adverse reactions to inactive ingredients added to medications, in 1985, the American Pediatric Academy's Committee on Drugs strongly urged our FDA to mandate labeling of all inactive ingredients in over-the-counter and prescription drugs. However, labeling of inactive ingredients remains voluntary while old and new adverse reactions continue to be reported. Today, many medical providers still think the side effects caused by inactive ingredients are irrelevant, even though many are known to cause the very symptoms their prescription medications are intended to cure (Committee on Drugs, 1997). The FDA's lax voluntary regulations are clearly inadequate; for example, (Committee on Drugs, 1997):

> Saccharin is present in drugs in substantial amounts. Ingestion of chewable aspirin or acetaminophen tablets in a school-age child can provide approximately the same amount of saccharin contained in one can of a diet soft drink. This amount, relative to the bodyweight of a child younger than 10 years, ingested for prolonged periods can be considered as "heavy use," as defined in a major large-scale FDA/ National Cancer Institute epidemiologic study. In this study, the heavy use of artificial sweeteners was associated with a significantly increased risk for the development of bladder cancer.
>
> Saccharin causes similar dermatologic reactions. Children with "sulfa" allergy should avoid medications made with saccharin.
>
> Studies found that medications containing saccharin most frequently caused pruritus and urticaria, followed by eczema, sensitivity to light, and chronic skin itchiness. Other reactions include wheezing, nausea, diarrhea, tongue blisters, tachycardia, fixed eruptions, headache, diuresis, and sensory neuropathy. Ingestion of saccharin-adulterated milk formula by infants was

associated with irritability, hypertonia, insomnia, muscle spasms causing back-arching, and weak eye muscles. Because of the paucity of data on the toxicity of saccharin in children, the American Medical Association has recommended limiting the intake of saccharin in young children and pregnant women.

Multiple sulfite compounds are "Generally Recognized as Safe" for use in foods and drugs. This status was revoked for raw fruits and vegetables, excluding potatoes, in 1986, after the FDA received reports of more than 250 cases of adverse reactions, including six deaths associated with the ingestion of sulfites in foods. Although primary exposure in children is through foods, serious reactions have occurred after oral and inhalational administration of sulfite-containing drugs. Signs and symptoms most frequently reported include wheezing, shortness of breath, and chest tightness in patients with known reactive airway disease. The incidence of sulfite sensitivity increases with age in severely asthmatic people. The presence of sulfites in anti-asthmatic medications is a concern; therefore, inhalers without sulfites can be prescribed. Nevertheless, avoiding foods containing sulfites through careful reading of packaged food labels and inquiry at restaurants as to their use of agents that contain sulfites can prevent reactions.

In 1972, President Nixon introduced the Environmental Protection Agency (EPA) to be responsible for the protection of our land and water from human activities.

In 1990 the Nutrition Labeling and Education Act (NLEA) was enacted by President George Bush Sr. This law gave the FDA the authority to require nutrition labeling of most foods regulated by their agency and to require that all nutrient content claims and health claims meet FDA regulations.

In the meantime, biotechnology continued to advance, but it was not until 1994 that genetically manipulated food was deregulated and allowed to be sold to Americans without consumer awareness. In 1996, the first genetically modified product, the Flavr Savr tomato, was sold to Americans without any warning that they contained DNA from seafood, bacteria, and antibiotics.

Individual states have since attempted to make labeling of GMO foods mandatory, but the 114th Congress in 2014 passed a federal law making it illegal for any state to mandate the labeling of GMO foods or ingredients. This was dubbed as the DARK Act, which stands for "Denying Americans the Right to Know."

So, who are our elected officials working for? The American people or the international food industry?

"The Farm Bill and other government actions contributed greatly to the crisis. It will take a grass-roots effort to return the balance in our food system. Recently efforts have sprung up, which are slowly turning the tide. These include organic farmers' markets, buying local, farm shares, organic home gardens, and a return to natural products such as raw milk, pastured eggs, and meat. Cooking and eating real food at home with our families cannot be emphasized enough in resolving these major issues" (Onusic, 2013).

It is evident that our elected officials play a very prominent role in food safety in the USA. So do food lobbyists in Washington, hence keeping abreast of what food labels tell us or do not reveal is something all consumers should be aware of.

Some basic information that may help you make healthy food choices are:

☺ Product Lookup Code (PLU) sticker found on all fresh produce may tell you more than you Realize

☺ What food labels tell us

☺ Which ingredients are regulated & how tell if you are the exception to its safety?

☺ Sneaky ways POB's can be deceiving

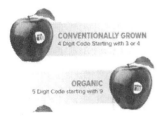

**Product Lookup Code (PLU) Sticker
on all Fresh Produce
Tells You More Than You Realize**

PLU codes are those tiny stickers you find stuck to most individual produce sold in supermarkets. The International Federation for Produce Standards (IFPS) is a global organization comprised of national produce associations from around the world. They're responsible for deciding which codes are assigned to which foods. There are currently 1,400 PLU codes used worldwide. The IFPS assigns codes using the 3000, 4000, 93000, and 94000 series. Each PLU is unique to its grower, but all are categorized by a specific type of produce.

The use of PLU codes is not mandated in the USA. This is the same kind of legislation as other food labeling, which is not mandatory. Most supermarkets use stickers to make inventory and pricing easier. Food labeling is completely voluntary, and retailers can label items as they choose. For example, many people are unaware that genetically modified vegetables are often labeled as *conventionally grown*.

There is no distinct PLU code for genetically modified produce. Many types of conventionally grown produce have genetically modified organisms (GMO) scientifically engineered into their produce. The added DNA can come from unrelated plants, animals, and microorganisms. Vegetarian consumers have no way of knowing whether animal DNA has been added to their vegetables and fruit. According to a 2013 report by the Grocery Manufacturers Association (Charles, 2013), as much as 80% percent of all foods sold in American contain GMOs.

Due to the increased production of GMO crops, cross-contamination has been difficult to control. Even when a label states Non-GMO, under current standards in the USA, these grain and crop production can still contain up to 10% GMO genes.

US legislators in 1994 passed laws that deemed all produce sold in the USA regardless of its origins are deemed raw and, therefore, automatically are GRAS. Bypassing such legislation, the FDA and USDA have not regulatory power over these crops.

With all this said, there is some universal information that comes from these PLU numbers. The first number tells consumers how that produce was grown. Organic produce always starts with #9 on the sticker. This means the grower complies with all of the rigid restrictions that qualify their product as organic. If you use the peels or zest of fruits in your home-baked foods, you will want only to use organic produce, because these are certified not to contain harmful pesticide residues.

Conventional produce begins with the numbers #3 or #4. These are unregulated produce that may contain genes from other plants, animals, microorganisms, and even medications such as antibiotics, vaccines and birth control, (Moss, 2010), (Whitwan, 2014). They may have glyphosate, dicamba, and other harmful chemical residues on them. Produce saturated in pesticides can be more harmful to some people than others; thereby sending your child to school with a #3 or #4 apple or other produce that your child will eat the skin, you may be inadvertently feeding your child harmful additives known to cause allergies, learning disabilities or other health conditions.

Also, vegans, vegetarians, and anyone with chronic health conditions should be aware that conventionally grown produce may not contain the same nutrients or composition as the organic variety. These unknown constituents can inadvertently affect prescribed medications or induce other health problems. A survey in the International Journal of Human Nutrition and Functional Medicine found that people who reduced or eliminated their consumption of GMO foods experienced an improvement in digestion, food sensitivities, and energy levels (Smith, 2017) in addition to feeling full quicker with less food and calories.

PLU codes have the technology to tell consumers:

- ✓ Exactly where produce is grown
- ✓ What seeds were used to grow that crop-- organic or conventional: If conventional seeds were used-- what specific animal, plant, and microbe DNA was genetically engineered into that produce?
- ✓ What chemicals have been applied, and how much residue remains on produce at the time of sale?
- ✓ Are there any consumers who should avoid that product for any reason?

Some producers already take advantage of this feature to promote the safety of their products. Consumers can look up their PLU code and get a lot of information about that fruit or vegetable. Even though the technology to provide this information is already used by other countries, legislators in the USA have not mandated producers to provide this information to consumers.

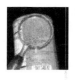 **What Food Labels Tell Us:**

The purpose of labels on food is *consumer awareness*. Produce have Product Lookup codes (PLU), whereas processed foods have labels.

Foods can be organic, natural, or genetically engineered. Whichever you prefer, labels should be providing sufficient information in terms that are easy to understand. Probably the most important part of any label is its serving size, nutrients, ingredients, and potential allergens.

- *A serving size* is the number of servings per packaged or container.
  - The information on the rest of the nutrient panel is based on each serving.
  - If the label states 4 servings in the package, the nutrient values listed describe each serving. If more than 1/4th of that package is consumed, then additional calories and other nutrients must be factored into your daily intake. For example: If that label states there are 4 servings per container and 100 calories per serving, eating the entire package will add up to 400 calories.
  - The same is true for all the other nutrients, including sugar. If a 14 oz can of peas is 2.5 servings and there is 6 gm of sugar per serving, then consuming the entire 14 oz can of peas will provide 15 gm of sugar.
  - Many processed foods that are packaged as a single serving can be misleading when they actually contain two or more servings. According to the Nutrition Labeling and Education Act (NLEA) of 1990, a food item in a relatively small container may be labeled as a single serving if the entire contents can "reasonably be expected to be consumed in a single-eating occasion."

  - However, there is often a discrepancy. Items to watch out for include: Large muffins that may state 160 calories but often contain two servings making the full muffin 320 calories; individual size ice cream containers that list calories as 150 but indicate it is 4 servings making the entire single-serving carton 600 calories.

- *Nutrients* are listed by the amount per serving and percentage of recommended daily intake.
  - In a previous chapter, I discussed the percentage of diet that should consist of 30% fat (9 calories per gram), 20 – 30% protein (4 calories per gram), and about 30 – 40% healthy carbohydrates (4 calories per gram). Nutrient panels on processed food list how many grams of each nutrient are in each serving. This is essential information for planning a balanced diet.
  - Nutrient panels that list '0' for most nutrients are considered to be empty calories.

- **Sugar** is the one exception on the nutrient panel: While other nutrients list *Daily Recommended Percentage*, food labels do not provide a daily recommended percentage for sugar content. This is because there is no minimum daily recommended amount; our body doesn't need sugar. According to the American Heart Association (AHA), the maximum amount of sugar anyone should eat in a day is:

  ☺ Men: 150 calories per day (37.5 grams or 9 teaspoons)
  ☺ Women: 100 calories per day (25 grams or 6 teaspoons)

  For example, an 8 oz can of cola have 25 gms of sugar, which is the maximum recommended amount of sugar from all sources for one day for women, whereas a 12 oz can contain 37.5 grams, which is the maximum amount for men.

- *Ingredients*
  o Food labels list ingredients in descending order from the greatest amount to the least. The most prevalent ingredient is first, and the least is listed last.
  o Exempt Ingredients can be misleading. Ingredients that constitute less than 2 percent can be listed in any order after the heading as "contains less than 2% of the following:"
  o The same ingredient may have multiple names used by the same or different manufactures
  o The ingredient lists can be a useful tool to figure out where unhealthy symptoms care to come from. Looking up additives that are in foods you consume regularly may have side-effects that are causing your poor health symptoms or making your symptoms worse.
- *Potential allergens* must be listed as a warning to those who may be allergic to specific ingredients.

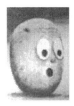

How are ingredients regulated?
How do you know if you are the exception?
Which ingredients will cause you harm?

There are three primary federal agencies responsible for the safety of food sold to consumers in America. Each is responsible for different aspects of the quality and processing of various foods and has multiple divisions within their department. These three agencies are"

- ✓ The Food and Drug Administration (FDA)
- ✓ The United States Department of Agriculture (USDA)
- ✓ The Environmental Protection Agency (EPA)

Each agency has its own website and is responsible for making the public aware of what products they approve and why including any limitations such as the maximum amount to safely consume. Registered Dietitians and medical professionals can help identify which foods specific individuals should avoid. A few concerns consumers should be aware of when evaluating the safety of specific additives, POB meat and plant products, medication, and pesticide residues include:

- ☺ What are the symptoms it can cause?
- ☺ What is the maximum amount a person can safely consume?
- ☺ Can medication or pesticide residue interact with my prescribed medications?
    - o Could uncontrolled diabetes, blood pressure, etc. be caused by specific meat or plant products that have medication or pesticide residue that makes my prescribed medication act erratically?

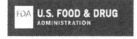

The FDA

"Many new techniques are being researched that will allow the production of additives in ways not previously possible. One approach is the use of biotechnology, which can use simple organisms to produce food additives. These additives are the same as food components found in nature.

In 1990, the FDA approved the first bioengineered enzyme, rennin, which traditionally had been extracted from calves' stomachs for use in making cheese. The following summary lists the types of common food ingredients, why they are used, and some examples of the names that can be found on product labels. Some additives are used for more than one purpose" (FDA, 2010).

"About 48 million people in the U.S. (1 in 6) get sick, 128,000 are hospitalized, and 3,000 die each year from foodborne diseases, according to recent data from the Centers for Disease Control and Prevention. This is a significant public health burden that is largely preventable. The FDA Food Safety Modernization Act of 2011 (FSMA) is transforming the nation's food safety system by shifting the focus from responding to foodborne illness to preventing it. Congress enacted FSMA in response to dramatic changes in the global food system and in our understanding of foodborne illness and its consequences, including the realization that preventable foodborne illness is both a significant public health problem and a threat to the economic well-being of the food system. FDA has finalized seven major rules to implement FSMA, recognizing that ensuring the safety of the food supply is a shared responsibility among many different points in the global supply chain for both human and animal food. The FSMA rules are designed to make clear specific actions that must be taken at each of these points to prevent contamination" (FDA, n.d).

For more information about the FDA, food additives, and food safety, go to www.fda.gov.

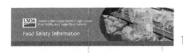 **USDA**

"What does 'mechanically separated meat or poultry' mean?" "If chicken is labeled 'fresh,' how can it be so rock hard?" "Does 'natural' mean 'raised without hormones'?" These are just some of the question's consumers

Rebekah S. Mead

have asked USDA's Meat and Poultry Hotline about words which may be descriptive of meat and poultry.

Can they be legally used on labels, and, if so, what are their definitions? Here from USDA's Food Safety and Inspection Service (FSIS) is a glossary of meat and poultry labeling terms. FSIS is the agency responsible for ensuring the truthfulness and accuracy in labeling of meat and poultry products. Knowing the meaning of labeling terms can make purchasing of meat and poultry products less confusing (USDA, 2006):

Meat and Poultry Labeling Terms	USDA Meat & Poultry Hotline 1-888-MPHotline (1-888-674-6854)
Basted or Self Basted	Bone-in poultry products that are injected or marinated with a solution containing butter or other edible fat, broth, stock or water plus spices, flavor enhancers, and other approved substances must be labeled as basted or self-basted. The maximum added weight of approximately a 3% solution before processing is included in the net weight on the label. The label must include a statement identifying the total quantity and common or usual name of all ingredients in the solution, e.g., "Injected with approximately 3% of a solution of -------------- (list of ingredients)."
Certified	The use of the terms "basted" or "self-basted" on boneless poultry products is limited to 8% of the weight of the raw poultry before processing.
Chemical Free Free-Range or Free-Roaming Fresh Poultry	The term "certified" implies that the USDA's Food Safety and Inspection Service and the Agriculture Marketing Service have officially evaluated a meat product for class, grade, or other quality characteristics (e.g., "Certified Angus Beef"). When used under other circumstances, the term must be closely associated with the name of the organization responsible for the "certification" process, e.g., "XYZ Company's Certified Beef."
Basted or Self Basted	The term is not allowed to be used on a label.
Certified	Producers must demonstrate to the Agency that the poultry has been allowed access to the outside.
Fresh Poultry	In August 1995, USDA/FSIS published a rule attempting to modify the definition of "fresh" to refer to poultry whose internal temperature has never been below 26 °F. That rule said poultry, whose internal temperature is between 26 °F and 0 °F, cannot be called "fresh" but must be called "hard-chilled" or "previously hard chilled." In January 1996, the final rule was published in the Federal Register. However, Congress did not appropriate money for enforcing the rule. On August 8, 1996, Congress asked FSIS to revise the final rule. FSIS has now amended the poultry product inspection regulations to prohibit the use of the term "fresh" on the labeling of raw poultry products whose internal temperature has ever been below 26 °F.

234

Also, labels of raw poultry products whose temperature has ever been below 26 °F, but above 0 °F, will not be required to bear any specific, descriptive labeling terms, including "hard chilled" or "previously hard chilled." To be in compliance with the revised rule, raw poultry products that are labeled as "fresh" but have ever had an internal temperature In August 1995 USDA/FSIS published a rule attempting to modify the definition of "fresh" to refer to poultry whose internal temperature has never been below 26 °F. That rule said poultry, whose internal temperature is between 26 °F and 0 °F, cannot be called "fresh" but must be called "hard-chilled" or "previously hard chilled."

In January 1996, the final rule was published in the Federal Register. However, Congress did not appropriate money for enforcing the rule. On August 8, 1996, Congress asked FSIS to revise the final rule. FSIS has below 26 °F will have to have the "fresh" designation deleted or removed from labeling on the package.

The final rule also sets a temperature tolerance for raw poultry products. The temperature of individual packages of raw poultry products labeled "fresh" can vary as much as 1°F below 26 °F within inspected establishments or 2 °F below 26 °F in commerce. This revised final rule appeared in the December 17, 1996, Federal Register and became effective 1 year later -- December 17, 1997.

Frozen Poultry Fryer-Roaster Turkey Halal and Zabiah Halal	The temperature of raw, frozen poultry is 0 °F or below.
Hen or Tom Turkey	Young, immature turkey usually less than 16 weeks of age of either sex.
Kosher	Products prepared by federally inspected meat packing plants identified with labels bearing references to "Halal" or "Zabiah Halal" must be handled according to Islamic law and under Islamic authority.
"Meat" Derived by Advanced Meat/Bone Separation and Meat Recovery Systems	The sex designation of "hen" (female) or "tom" (male) turkey is optional on the label and is an indication of size rather than the tenderness of a turkey.
Mechanically Separated Meat	"Kosher" may be used only on the labels of meat and poultry products prepared under Rabbinical supervision.
Mechanically Separated Poultry	The definition of "meat" was amended in December 1994 to include as "meat" product derived from advanced meat/bone separation machinery, which is comparable in appearance, texture, and composition to meat trimmings and similar meat products derived by hand. The products produced by advanced meat recovery (AMR) machinery can be labeled using terms associated with the hand-deboned product, e.g., pork trimmings and ground pork. The AMR machinery cannot grind, crush or pulverize bones to remove edible meat tissue, and bones must emerge essentially

	intact. The meat produced in this manner can contain no more than 150 milligrams of calcium per 100 grams product.
Natural	A product containing no artificial ingredient or added color and is only minimally processed (a process which does not fundamentally alter the raw product) may be labeled natural. The label must explain the use of the term natural (such as - no added colorings or artificial ingredients; minimally processed.)
No Hormones (pork or poultry)	Hormones are not allowed in raising hogs or poultry. Therefore, the claim "no hormones added" cannot be used on the labels of pork or poultry unless it is followed by a statement that says, "Federal regulations prohibit the use of hormones."
No Hormones (beef)	The term "no hormones administered" may be approved for use on the label of beef products if sufficient documentation is provided to the Agency by the producer showing no hormones have been used in raising the animals.
No Antibiotics (red meat and poultry)	The terms "no antibiotics added" may be used on labels for meat or poultry products if sufficient documentation is provided by the producer to the Agency, demonstrating that the animals were raised without antibiotics.
Organic	For information about the National Organic Program and use of the term "organic" on labels, refer to these factsheets from the USDA Agricultural Marketing Service: • Organic Food Standards and Labels: The Facts • Labeling and Marketing Information
Oven Prepared Oven Ready Young Turkey	The product is fully cooked and ready to eat.

USDA STANDARDS OF ORGANIC: CHECK THE LABEL

The U.S. Department of Agriculture (USDA) established an organic certification program that requires all organic foods to meet strict government standards. These standards regulate how such foods are grown, handled, and processed. The USDA also has guidelines on how organic foods are described on product labels (Drugs.com, 2018):

☺ **100 percent organic.** This description is used on certified organic fruits, vegetables, eggs, meat, or other single-ingredient foods. It may also be used on multi-ingredient foods if all of the ingredients are certified organic, excluding salt and water. These may have a USDA seal.

☺ **Organic.** If a multi-ingredient food is labeled organic, at least 95 percent of the ingredients are certified organic, excluding salt and water. The nonorganic items must be from a USDA list of approved additional ingredients. These also may have a USDA seal.

☺ **Made with organic.** If a multi-ingredient product has at least 70 percent certified organic ingredients, it may have a "made with organic" ingredients label. For example, a breakfast cereal might be labeled "made with organic oats." The ingredient list must identify what ingredients are organic. These products may not carry a USDA seal.

☺ **Organic ingredients.** If less than 70 percent of a multi-ingredient product is certified organic, it may not be labeled as organic or carry a USDA seal. The ingredient list can indicate which ingredients are organic.

$EPA United States Environmental Protection Agency **The Environmental Protection Agency (EPA)**

The EPA is responsible for the health and safety of our land, water, animals, and human life. It monitors the safety of pesticides in use and analysis new one prior to use.

"The U.S. Environmental Protection Agency (EPA) has a critical role in food security and safety within the United States, in areas such as food safety, water quality, and pesticide applicator training. The EPA is responsible for ensuring that the American public is protected from potential health risks posed by eating foods that have been treated with pesticides. The Agency is responsible both for the registration of new pesticides before they can be marketed and the re-registration of older pesticides to ensure that they meet current scientific standards. EPA uses the National Research Council's four-step process for human health risk assessment: Hazard Identification, Dose-Response Assessment, Exposure Assessment, and Risk Assessment.

Since the passage of the Food Quality Protection Act of 1996, the EPA is undertaking a comprehensive review of tolerances for pesticide residues in food. The focus of the review included an increase in protection for infants and children as well as other vulnerable groups. Progress of this review can be found at the following Web site: http://www.epa.gov/pesticides/tolerance/ reassessment.htm.

A pesticide is any agent used to kill or control undesired insects, weeds, rodents, fungi, bacteria, or other organisms.

Pesticides are classified according to their function: insecticides control insects, rodenticides control rodents; herbicides control weeds; and fungicides control fungi, mold, and mildew. Herbicides are the most widely used type of pesticide in agriculture. Chemical pest control plays a significant role in modern agriculture and has contributed to dramatic increases in crop yields over the past four decades for most field, fruit, and vegetable crops.

Pesticides cause illness in human adults with even more severe symptoms in children and pets if absorbed on contact, inhaled, or eaten. The EPA sets maximum residue limits on the amount of pesticide residue that can lawfully remain in or on each treated food commodity. EPA considers the toxicity, amount and frequency of pesticide application, and how much of the pesticide (and or pesticide residue) remains in or on food. An added margin of safety ensures that residues remaining in foods are many times lower than amounts that could actually cause adverse health effects. The Food and Drug Administration (FDA), which monitors domestically produced and imported foods traveling in interstate commerce except for meat, poultry, and some egg products, enforces the pesticide tolerances set by the EPA.

Integrated Pest Management (IPM) uses an array of pest control methods to achieve better results with the least disruption (harm) to the environment including cultivating pest-resistant plants, adjusting planting times to avoid pest infestation, using beneficial or predatory insects (ladybugs), station traps containing phenomes (sex hormones) to remove fertile adult insects, destroying nesting areas, removing leaf clutter etc. Studies suggest that IPM techniques generally increase crop yields and economic profits while reducing the use of chemical pesticides. Modern biotechnology has enabled the production of new plant-pesticides. For example, new types of agricultural plants that have been altered to produce proteins toxic to insects that destroy crops. Such plant-pesticides reduce the need for conventional pesticide applications, thereby reducing production costs as well as risks to workers and non-target insects. For additional information, please visit EPA's pesticide programs:

- http://www.epa.gov/pesticides/ US Farmer and Rancher Alliance
- http://www.fooddialogues.com/foodsource/pesticides-fertilizer-herbicides" (Lwstl.org, 2018).

The EPA website contains a lot of information about the safety of chemicals approved for use that can help identify who is most at risk of exposure. Below are a few guidelines that can be found at the EPA website. (EPA, 2019):

EPA Guidelines

The following tables includes guidance documents, handbooks, framework documents, standard operating procedures (SOPs), and other related materials developed by EPA for human health risk assessments.

Show 10 entries   Search:

Title	Year	Keywords
A Framework for Assessing Health Risk of Environmental Exposures to Children	2006	Children
A Review of the Reference Dose and Reference Concentration Processes	2002	Reference
A Summary of General Assessment Factors for Evaluating the Quality of Scientific and Technical Information	2003	Factors
Acute oral toxicity up-and-down procedure	2002	Pesticides, Oral
Advances in genetic toxicology and integration of in vivo testing into standard repeat dose studies		Pesticides, Toxicology
Alpha2u-Globulin: Association with Chemically Induced Renal Toxicity and Neoplasia in the Male Rat	1991	Toxicity
Alternate testing framework for classification of eye irritation potential of EPA-regulated pesticide products	2015	Pesticides, Classification
Assessment of Thyroid Follicular Cell Tumors	1998	
Available information on assessing exposure from pesticides in food—A User's Guide	2007	Pesticides, Food
Benchmark Dose Technical Guidance	2012	BMDS

Sneaky ways POB Foods can fool us:

Information should be clear and accurate using familiar terms, but sometimes labels are misleading. For instance: Fats may be listed as "partially hydrogenated oil" in the list of ingredients on a label. If the nutrition facts on a label say, the product has "0 g trans-fat," that doesn't necessarily mean it has no trans-fats. It could have up to half a gram of trans fats per serving. This means that a serving size on 10 potato chips has 0.5 grams of trans-fat and the entire bag has 3.5 servings, eating the entire bag of chips may have added up to 1.75 grams of trans-fat.

Another way food manufacturer misleads consumers is by using unfamiliar terms or listing the same ingredient using multiple different names to make the additive appear to be in lesser quantity than it really is. For instance, if a product is mostly high fructose corn syrup (HFCS), instead of listing it as the number one ingredient, which may cause many consumers to choose another brand, the manufacturer may list it three different ways to make it appear as though the undesired ingredient is only the fifth-highest amount. In doing so, they list HFCS as the fifth ingredient, corn starch as the sixth ingredient and corn syrup as the seventh ingredient. They are all broken down in our bodies the way to produce the same simple sugar.

Monosodium gluconate (MSG) is an ingredient in many additives that consumers trying to avoid MSG may not be aware of. Any consumers who suffer from migraines and other symptoms related to MSG consumption should avoid all ingredients which contain MSG, (See chapter 9: MSG)

Occasionally, labels on food can be downright wrong. "Despite being regulated by the FDA and the U.S. Department of Agriculture, food manufacturers can get away with adding confusing or deceptive information to the labels. This may be done inadvertently, but often it's done with the specific intention of making you think the food is better for you than it actually is. Some foods that claim to include healthy ingredients actually don't contain them, or only contain them in minuscule amounts" (Sixwise.com, 2009).

I recently experienced this at my local grocery store. I usually buy a butter product that substitutes less than half its organic cream with olive oil. My usual brand contains only three ingredients: Cream, olive oil, and salt. I bake with 100% butter, but for meals where I add butter, I serve the combination of butter-olive oil in an effort to reduce the animal fat in my diet. As I was doing my weekly shopping, next to the tub of butter-olive oil in the dairy section, I saw a competitor brand that boldly stated on its label, "made with olive oil." It was half the price of what I usually buy, so I picked it up and looked at its ingredients: #1 ingredient was water, then soy oil, canola oil, and a bunch of preservatives and other additives including corn syrup. There was no cream in it, which is where butter comes from, and the very last of about ten ingredients was olive oil. The front label emphasized this substitute butter was made with olive oil, but then the ingredient panel lowest it was the last ingredient, which indicated it was a minute amount of olive oil. It was mostly GMO soy products.

Organic and Natural do not mean the same thing (Drugs.com, 2018):
Another term that can be misleading is the term "Natural." Natural and organic are not interchangeable terms. In general, "natural" on a food label means that it has no artificial colors, flavors, or preservatives. It does not refer to the methods or materials used to produce the food ingredients.

An example of a standard food label that may confuse natural with organic labels is the guidelines for certified organic beef. Organic has a number of requirements, such as access to pasture during a minimum 120-day grazing season and no growth hormones. Whereas, the labels "free-range" or "hormone-free," while they must be used truthfully, do not indicate a farmer followed all guidelines for organic certification (Drugs.com, 2018).

The term all-natural actually has no nutritional meaning whatsoever and isn't regulated by the FDA. What is considered natural can be ambiguous; for example, transglutaminase occurs naturally in goats and pigs, but when used to glue meat from different animals to form a steak or roast (P, 2018) those products did not occur naturally in nature.

What is natural isn't always safe. Products with the 'natural' labeling are not required by law to contain only natural ingredients. "Consumers think of words like 'safe' and 'good for me' when they think of natural, but across the board, from prescription drugs to food products, many of these natural claims are misleading at best," (Food Editor, 2019).

"Free from..." is another phrase that can be used to misrepresent food. The FDA allows food manufacturers to round to zero any ingredient that accounts for less than 0.5 grams per serving. So, while a product may claim to be "GMO-free," "gluten-free," "Sugar-free," or "alcohol-free,' it can legally contain up to 0.5 grams per serving. While this may seem like an insignificant amount, depending on the ingredient, it may be enough to cause a reaction when:

- Consumed in multiple servings or in various foods throughout the day
- Consumed frequently over time this small fraction can add up

Case in point, many food products that claim to have no dangerous trans-fats list partially hydrogenated oil in their ingredients label, which the World Health Organization is trying to eliminate because of its harm to health (WHO, 2018). Partially hydrogenated oil creates trans fats, so these labels may be taking advantage of the rounding to zero option. "If there's less than 0.5 gram of trans fats per serving, the food manufacturer may round down to zero" (Sixwise.com, 2009).

Bottom line: To make healthy food choices, American consumers must become aware of the laws that standardize food labels. What we chose to put into our body can make the difference between being healthy or sick.

Key Points

♣ Food laws vary from country to country. Some foods and food additives are known to be harmful in other countries are GRAS in the USA

♣ More than 130 other nations have signed the Cartagena Act, which requires POB to be proven safe to humans and the environment prior to its sale. American legislators have not signed this

♣ Many derivatives from GMO soy are in most processed food in the supermarket. The food industry has replaced much of the American diet with imitation food made from GMO soy: Soymilk, soy butter, soy cheese, soy meat, soy oil in peanut butter, and salad dressing.

♣ A well-balanced diet cannot depend on one plant, and doing so will inevitably cause malnutrition because every human requires at least ninety different nutrients that come from a variety of natural plants and animals. A healthy diet consists of a variety of plant and animal foods.

♣ The FDA's lax voluntary regulations are clearly inadequate; for example, Saccharin is present in drugs in substantial amounts. Ingestion of chewable aspirin or acetaminophen tablets in a school-age child can provide approximately the same amount of saccharin contained in one can of a diet soft drink. This amount, relative to the body weight, can be considered as "heavy use." Research showed that the heavy use of artificial sweeteners was associated with a significantly increased risk for the development of bladder cancer.

♣ Saccharin causes similar dermatologic reactions. Children with "sulfa" allergy should avoid medications made with saccharin.

♣ The sticker on each piece of fruit we buy in the supermarket is called the Product Look Up code (PLU). The first number tells us whether the product is organic, #9, or non-organic, #3 and #4

♣ If you use the peels or zest of fruits in your home-baked foods, you will want only to use organic produce, because these are certified not to contain harmful pesticide residues.

♣ Labels can be misleading; therefore, it is the consumer's responsibility to learn how the food each person consumes is cultivated and what effects may those foods have on his or her health

♣ When looking at a label, look at how many servings are in each package. Calories and nutrients are based on each serving, not the entire package

♣ Three government agencies provide oversight for food safety in the USA; each has informative websites that help American consumers make healthier and more informed decisions about the foods they eat

♣ Beware that food additive and chemical residues may interact with prescribed medications or may cause health problems in some people

♣ Food producers may use multiple names for the same product; therefore, if trying to avoid a specific additive, become familiar with all of its alias.'

♣ The reason labels do not give a percentage of recommended daily allowance for sugar is because there is none. Our body does not need sugar

References

Charles, D. (2013). *How American food companies Go GMO-free In a GMO world.* Retrieved from NPR: https://www.npr.org/sections/thesalt/2014/02/04/269479079/how-american-food-companies-go-gmo-free-in-a-gmo-world

Drugs.com. (2018). *Organic Food: Are they Safer to Eat.* Retrieved from Drugs.com: https://www.drugs.com/mca/organic-foods-are-they-safer-more-nutritious

EPA. (2019). *EPA guidelines.* Retrieved from US Environmental Protection Agency: https://19january2017snapshot.epa.gov/risk/risk-assessment-guidelines_.html

FDA. (2010). *Overview of food ingredients, additives, and colors .* Retrieved from US Food and Drug Administration: https://www.fda.gov/food/food-ingredients-packaging/overview-food-ingredients-additives-colors#types

FDA. (n.d). *Food safety modernization act.* Retrieved from Food and Drug Administration: https://www.fda.gov/food/guidance-regulation-food-and-dietary-supplements/food-safety-modernization-act-fsma

Food Editor. (2019). *Food nutrition labels: Six "catches" you need to know.* Retrieved from Street Directory: https://www.streetdirectory.com/food_editorials/health_food/healthy_eating/food_nutrition_labels_six_catches_you_need_to_know.html

GMO Science. (2018). *The Impossible Burger:Boon or risk to health and the environment.* Retrieved from GMO Science: https://www.gmoscience.org/impossible-burger-boon-risk-health-environment/

Lwstl.org. (2018). *Food safety and pesticides.* Retrieved from Environmental Protection Agency: http://www.lwvstl.org/files/Food_Safety_and_Pesticides.pdf

Moss, L. (2010). *Banana vaccines.* Retrieved from Mother Nature : https://www.mnn.com/green-tech/research-innovations/photos/12-bizarre-examples-of-genetic-engineering/banana-vaccines#top-desktop

P. K. (2018). *Meat glue: What is it? What should you know?* Retrieved from Delishably: https://delishably.com/food-industry/Meat-Glue-What-It-Is-And-What-You-Should-Know

Rainer. (2018). *Why the Impossible Burger cannot be stopped.* Retrieved from Meat Alternatives: http://www.grubstreet.com/2018/04/impossible-foods-gets-more-funding-and-washington-lobbyist.html

Sixwise.com. (2009). *Food nutrition labels: Six catches you need to know.* Retrieved from Sixwise.com: http://www.sixwise.com/newsletters/05/11/02/food-nutrition-labels-six-catches-you-need-to-know.htm

Smith, J. (2017). Survey reports improved health after avoiding genetically modified foods. *Institute for Responsible Technology. International Journal of Human Nutrition and Functional Medicine.*

Starr-Hull, J. (2014). *Aspartame approval history.* Retrieved from JanetHull.com: http://www.janethull.com/newsletter/0412/aspartame_approval_history_1.php

Whitwan, R. (2014). *Genetically engineered super-banana could save millions of lives.* Retrieved from Extremetech.com: https://www.extremetech.com/extreme/184435-genetically-engineered-super-banana-could-save-millions-of-lives

WHO. (2018). *WHO plans to eliminate industrially-produced trans-fatty acids from global food supply.* Retrieved from The World Health Organization

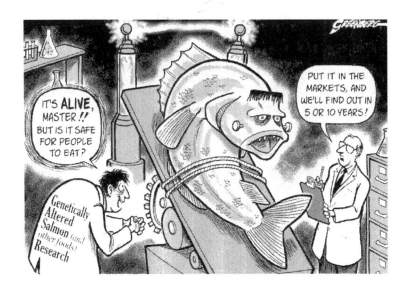

Chapter 9

What's Eating You - Food Reference Manual
Be Aware: Food, Food Additives & Other POB's have Side Effects
&
Avoid Those That Make You Sick

There are thousands of food additives and chemicals in food sold in the USA today, in addition to all the other kinds of POB used to alter organic plants and animals. And, the FDA GRAS standard is like the adage: It may harm all of the people some of the time, and some of the people all of the time, but it won't harm all of the people all of the time; therefore, any food or additive that does not harm everyone all of the time, is, by FDA standards, generally recognized as generally safe and legal to put into food sold to American consumers.

With so many alterations made to our food and new technology-foods added almost monthly without our knowledge, is it any wonder why new diseases with no cures in sight have quadrupled the cost of healthcare in

America? The best we Americans can do at this point is to become aware of what we are eating and make better-informed decisions. When symptoms of poor health occur, look at the foods we consumed recently or regularly. Do any of the ingredients listed on the labels cause those symptoms? If unsure, look them up individually on the internet.

There are enormous amounts of Evidence-Based Research (EBR) linking various food additives to the increase in violence, mental illness, and chronic physical conditions. These chemically induced health conditions place a heavy financial burden on our nation. Untested and unregulated compounds are added to the American food supply each year, of which many have several names for the same additive. All of which is making it impossible to know what we are consuming that is causing our health problems. With no mention of how much of each ingredient, we also have no way of knowing when we have eaten or drank a toxic amount.

There is accumulating evidence implementing the high intake of food additives in conjunction with a poor balance of nutrients is unnecessarily placing individuals at risk for organ failures, bone loss, obesity, cancer, alterations in microbiota, irritable bowel conditions and many other health conditions. In other words, food additives in our food, combined with a diet low in nutrients, are causing preventable illnesses that increase our need for medical care. Preventable chronic diseases are expensive, and they detract from the quality of our lives.

Ways that chemicals affect our food and prescribed medications include:

- ☹ Bioavailability: Impair our enzymes, hormones, and neurotransmitters in ways that prevent optimal absorption of nutrients
- ☹ Impair our body's ability to produce high-quality hormones, enzymes, and neurotransmitters
- ☹ Damage our healthy microbiota
- ☹ Damage to our hormones
- ☹ Overwork our filtering systems: Our kidneys and liver
- ☹ Cause damage to our brain- our command center
- ☹ Contradict the effects of medications
- ☹ Counter the effects of nutrients

Considering all of the evidence-based research about the affect's additives have on health, there is a need for a food reference manual that helps American consumers understand what additives do and what is the maximum recommended intake. Most consumers are not aware that a safe dose is often one-serving in one food containing that ingredient. For example, carrageenan and high fructose in ice cream are generally recognized as safe when consuming one portion daily in one type of food such as ice cream, which is usually ½ cup. Therefore, consuming any other products containing these ingredients on the same day may be consuming toxic levels. Other processed foods that may contain these two ingredients are A can of soda, cheese, two tablespoons of ketchup, or one tablespoon of salad dressing.

If American officials are going to continue to approve food additives that have the potential to harm our health, then American consumers need an efficient and easy way to understand those risks. For instance, because almost every processed food contains some form of GMO soy, then we need to know what is a safe amount of GMO soy to consume daily and what are the potential health risks. For every POB product, Americans need a food reference manual that explicitly tells us:

- ☺ Alternate names and aliases (a.k.a.)
- ☺ What is a safe dose
- ☺ Additional information: What research says
- ☺ Do one or more other countries ban it?
- ☺ What are the potential side effects
- ☺ Who should avoid it

If taking medication for specific conditions, those consumers should avoid all additives that can cause those symptoms. For example, people taking medication for anxiety should avoid any additive that is an excitotoxin and neurotoxic. Anyone taking medicines for heart disease should avoid foods that can cause heart disease. Also, anyone taking medication for muscle weakness, which entails shortness of breath and difficulty swallowing, because our lungs and digestive system use muscle, should avoid additives that cause muscle weakness.

Every American should beware that if every processed food you eat for breakfast, lunch, and dinner, and each snack in between, contains the same additives or chemicals, you may be consuming toxic levels that can be causing all of your health problems. Education about nutrition and how foods affect health should begin in elementary school.

Ultimately, your health is your responsibility. After all, you are what you eat!

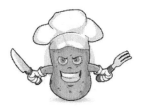

Aspartame

Alternate Names: Aspartame (APM), NutraSweet, SugarTwin, Equal, Canderel; In medication, it may be listed as phenylalanine

Purpose: Low calorie synthetic artificial sweetener. Approved as a flavor enhancer.

Nutritional Value: None

Acceptable Daily Intake (ADI): FDA states 50 mg per 2 Kg (2.2 lb.) of body weight per day.

It is found in At least 600 medications. It is in many low-calorie foods and beverages.

Additional Information

When digested, aspartame breaks down into three components: aspartic acid, phenylalanine, and methanol (wood alcohol):

1. Aspartic Acid (FDA, 2018), (Hathaway, 2017):
   - Aids in the breakdown of amino acids that help form enzymes used by the body
   - Chronic use can lead to leptin and/or insulin resistance
     - Elevated levels may cause obesity, diabetes, high cholesterol, and high blood pressure

2. Phenylalanine (NIH, 2017)(American Cancer Society, 2014). (FDA, 2018):
   - Is an amino acid derived from protein and some artificial sweeteners
   - Some people are born with a rare genetic disorder called phenylketonuria (PKU). These individuals cannot produce enough of the enzyme needed to break down phenylalanine. If untreated, it can lead to learning disabilities and other serious health problems
   - Aspartame may cause birth defects when consumed during pregnancy

3. Methanol (wood alcohol):

- Is filter by the liver
- Low toxicity in humans when consumed in small amounts
- Very small amounts occur naturally in fruit juices, whereas a little higher level occurs in fermented alcohol beverages
- Consumption of large amounts can cause damage to the Central Nervous System (CNS). Large amounts can affect vision and coordination
- May inhibit or increase the effect of medications prescribed for CNS conditions

Hyman J. Roberts, M.D., F.A.C.P., F.C.C.P., author of *Protecting Mankind,* was a medical provider and a scientist investigating poisons in our food and environment. His research identified aspartame as a chemical trigger for Parkinson's Disease. In 1995 the FDA published a list of 92 reactions to this toxin from over 10,000 volunteered consumer complaints. Dr. Roberts prepared a comprehensive 1,038-page medical text: *Aspartame Disease, An Ignored Epidemic*, including hundreds of patient histories, instructions for doctors, absolute evidence to Protect Mankind from a poison most Americans consume and by which they are slowly damaged or destroyed. The toxin is ingested in minute cumulative doses, bringing diverse and disperse symptoms, difficult for most doctors to diagnose especially since the FDA says it is safe, (Martini, 2008)

"Lean and Hankey's editorial on the effects of aspartame and health gives this artificial sweetener a clean bill of health. However, it seems they have ignored or dismissed a wealth of evidence, which shows that aspartame can provoke a wide range of symptoms. Studies (a total of 91) that attest to aspartame's potential for harm can be found in an online review of peer-reviewed literature. This review is particularly worrying as it shows that, although 100% of industry-funded studies conclude that aspartame is safe, 92% of independently funded studies have found that aspartame has the potential for adverse effects," (Briffa, 2005).

Parkinson's disease is a common central nervous system disorder that mainly affects the elderly population. It is believed Parkinson's disease is caused by a lack of dopamine, which is a chemical neurotransmitter responsible for controlling muscle movement. When dopamine levels are reduced, nerve endings cannot properly send movement messages, and muscle function is impaired. The scientific community regularly studies various food and beverage ingredients to determine if it has an effect on Parkinson's disease, and initial studies suggest the artificial sweetener aspartame has little to no effect on this nervous system disorder.

Aspartame is a synthetic artificial sweetener, frequently used in foods, medications, and beverages. This review examines research published between 2000 and 2016 on both the safe dosage and higher-than-recommended dosages and presents a concise synthesis of current trends. Many people consume a higher amount of aspartame than the recommended dose by consuming many servings (supersize soda in addition to consuming products that contain this ingredient). Since aspartame consumption is on the rise, the safety of this sweetener should be revisited. The existing animal studies and the limited human studies suggest that aspartame and its metabolites may disrupt the oxidant/antioxidant balance, induce oxidative stress, and damage cell membrane integrity, potentially affecting a variety of cells and tissues and causing a deregulation of cellular function, ultimately leading to systemic inflammation. Chronic use of aspartame can cause (Chaudhary, 2017):

- ✓ Increase blood clotting
- ✓ Inflammation and damage to the liver
- ✓ Inflammation and damage to kidneys
- ✓ Impair heart function
- ✓ Impair immune system
- ✓ Impair brain function
- ✓ Alter microbiota in such a way that affects the health of other organs

Banned in one or more other countries: Yes

Potential Side-effects (Choudhary, 2017) (Wulaningsih, 2017) (Abhilash, 2014) (Gray, 1996); if you experience any of these, you may want to avoid aspartame:

Anxiety	Kidney inflammation
Birth defects	Kidney damage
Breathing difficulties	Learning disability

Clotting, increase	Leptin resistance
Dementia	Nausea
Depression	Neurologic diseases
Diabetes	Oxidative stress
Diarrhea	Rash
Insomnia: Sleep disturbance	Seizures
Insulin resistance	Stress
Irritability; Moodiness	Visual changes
Increase Appetite	Vomiting

Anyone taking medications for any of the above symptoms or have the following conditions may want to avoid food and medications that contain this ingredient:

✓ Taking medications to treat any of the above symptoms such as anti-anxiety/depression medications, insulin or blood thinners
✓ Moodiness: Uncontrollable anger, anxiety, depression and/or violent behavior
✓ Dementia
✓ Learning disorders: Hyperactivity; Attention Deficit Hyperactivity Disorder (ADHD)
✓ Metabolic syndrome = Diabetes + Heart disease
✓ Neurological diseases such as Parkinson's and Gillian Barrett

REFERENCES

Abhilash, M. A. (2014). Chronic Effect of Aspartame on Ionic Homeostasis and Monoamine Neurotransmitters in the Rat Brain. *Int Journal of Toxicology*, 332-341.

Briffa, J. (2005). Aspartame and its effects on health. *British Medical Journal, 330(7486)*, 309–310.

Choudhary, A. L. (2017). Neurophysiological symptoms and aspartame: What is the connection? *Nutritional Neuroscience 21(5)*, 306-316.

Committee on Drugs. (1997). Inactive" Ingredients in Pharmaceutical Products: Update. *American Academy of Pediatrics; 99 (2)*, 268-278.

Gray, D. (1996). *Summary of adverse reactions attributed to aspartame.* Department of Health & Human Services; FDA.

Martini, B. (2008). *FDA reports- from 1995 to 1998- aspartame.* Retrieved from Mission Possible World Health International: http://www.mpwhi.com/fda_aspartame_reports.htm

NIH. (2017). *Phenylalanine.* Retrieved from National Institute of Health / US Library of Medicine / Genetic Home Reference: Phenylketonuria (commonly known as PKU) is an inherited disorder that increases the levels of a substance called phenylalanine in the blood. Phenylalanine is a building block of proteins (an amino acid) that is obtained through the diet. It is found in al

Wulaningsih, W. V. (2017). Investigating nutrition and lifestyle factors as determinants of abdominal obesity: an environment-wide study. *Int Journal on Obesity 41(2)*, 340-347.

Carrageenan

Alternate names (a.k.a.): Algas, Algue Rouge Marine, Ammonium Carrageenan, Calcium Carrageenan, Carrageenan gum, Chondrus Extract, Carrageen, Carrageenin, Carragenano, Carragenina, Chondrus crispus, Chondrus Extract, Euchema species, Red Marine Algae, Sodium Carrageenan or Potassium Carrageenan
Products containing carrageenan may be labeled as "natural," because it is derived from red seaweed.

Purpose: Widely used in the food industry as a binder and for its gelling, thickening, and stabilizing properties. Its main application is in dairy and meat products. Dairy products diluted with water can be thickened with carrageenan to improve texture and elasticity.

Products it is found in: Ice cream, chocolate milk, sherbet, jam, jelly, cheese, cheese spread, dressings, crackers, pastries, custard, evaporated milk, whipped cream, infant formula, soymilk, Tofu, pet food, medication, toothpaste, and weight loss products, (WHO, 2015), (WebMD, 2019).

Nutritional Value: None (WHO, 2015)

Daily Allowance: Due to its effects on the gut (digestive system), the maximum amount is estimated at 1100–1300 mg/kg body weight per day [2.2 kg = 1 lb.]

Additional Information:

Extracted from a variety of red seaweed (WHO, 2015)

"Potential effects of carrageenan in infants arise from direct action on the intestinal tract. A maximum of 0.1% is recommended in infant formula due to its risk for intestinal irritation" (WHO, 2015).

"Carrageenan has been determined to be safe as a food additive by the FDA, although some concern exists about its safety in infant formula; Europe authorities do not allow carrageenan in infant formulas" (Drugs.com, 2018).

"Animal studies repeatedly show that food-grade carrageenan in pet foods cause gastrointestinal inflammation and higher rates of intestinal lesions, ulcerations, and even malignant tumors" (Thixton, 2015).

"Individuals who have suffered for years from undiagnosed gastrointestinal symptoms -abdominal bloating, spastic colon, irritable bowel syndrome, and diagnosed diseases, such as ulcerative colitis- often find relief when they eliminate carrageenan from their diet" (Cornucopia Institute, 2016).

One survey respondent wrote: "Before I knew about carrageenan, I suffered tremendous stomach cramps, body aches and extreme bloating from eating certain foods, sandwich meat, ice cream, etc. My symptoms would last for a minimum of 24 hours, sometimes lasting for 48 hours. I had several exploratory procedures done to see if I had a blockage somewhere in my intestinal tract. I started to record a food journal and a list of ingredients of everything I ate and suddenly discovered my symptoms were caused solely by carrageenan" (Cornucopia Institute, 2016).

"Another survey respondent wrote: "Since eliminating carrageenan, I have had no problems with stomach cramps, body aches, or extreme bloating. I am extremely careful not to ingest even the smallest amount, as it will cause me hours of suffering. I am extremely strict about the products I purchase, and after having researched the terrible effects of this awful ingredient, I have taken extra precautions that my four children do not ingest anything that contains carrageenan" (Cornucopia Institute, 2016).

Carrageenan exposure alone led to glucose intolerance after only six days. Carrageenan, in combination with the high-fat diet, increased non-HDL cholesterol, glucose levels, leptin resistance, and increased inflammation of blood vessels and the intestinal colon. The results of this study indicate that carrageenan exposure in the typical western-diet may exacerbate the harmful effects of the high-fat diet and contribute to the development of diabetes and atherosclerotic disease in the general population (Bhattacharyya, 2015).

"Carrageenan (CGN) is GRAS for the entire human population. Yet, numerous contradicting indications and mechanistic studies support the controversy over the long-term effects of CGN intake in humans. The effects of CGN on predisposed populations, such as Crohn's or ulcerative colitis patients, or liable populations, e.g., infants or pregnant women, have not been addressed by rigorous studies. Revisiting the evidence on the beneficial and deleterious effects of CGN intake indicates that science has yet to exclude the possibility that long-term exposure to increasing levels of CGN in the human diet may compromise human health and well-being. Over time, CGN can have an accumulating effect that resemble symptoms of chronic low-grade inflammation in obesity, diabetes, and metabolic syndrome (Lasselin, 2014) (Pereira, 2014)" (Sclomet, 2018).

FDA Approved: The food additive carrageenan may be safely used in food in accordance with prescribed conditions and food to specific conditions. This food additive is intended for use in the amount necessary for an emulsifier, stabilizer, or thickener in foods, except for those standardized foods that do not provide for such use. To assure safe use of the additive, the label and labeling of the additive shall bear the name of the additive, carrageenan (FDA, 2018).

Banned in one or more other countries: Yes

Potential Side-Effects:

Allergies	Inflammation of vessels
Atherosclerosis	Intestinal cancer
Abdominal cramps	Intestinal inflammation
Bloating	Intestinal Lesions
Diabetes	Intestinal ulcerations
Diarrhea, urgent	Leptin resistance
Flatus / Gas	Intestinal Lesions

Glucose intolerance

Irritable Bowel Syndrome

High non-HDL cholesterol

Metabolic syndrome

Anyone taking medications for any of the above symptoms or have the following conditions may want to avoid food and medications that contain this ingredient:

- ✓ Irritable Bowel Syndrome or disease
- ✓ Ulcerative colitis / Crohns disease
- ✓ Bloating and gas pains after meals
- ✓ High Cholesterol
- ✓ Stomach ulcers, lesions or cancer

REFERENCES

Bhattacharyya, S. F. (2015). Journal of Diabetes Res. Exposure to common food additive carrageenan alone leads to fasting hyperglycemia and in combination with high-fat diet, exacerbates glucose intolerance and hyperlipidemia without effect on weight — *Journal of Diabetes Res.*

Cornucopia Institute. (2016). *Carrageenan: New Studies Reinforce Link to Inflammation, Cancer, and Diabetes.* Retrieved from Cornucopia Institute: https://www.cornucopia.org/wp-content/uploads/2016/04/CarageenanReport-2016.pdf

Drugs.com. (2018). *Carrageenan.* Retrieved from Drugs.com: https://www.drugs.com/inactive/carrageenan-208.html

FDA. (2018). *Sec. 172.620: Carrageenan.* Silver Springs, MD: Food and Drug Administration: Code of Federal Regulations Title 21 v. 3.

Lasselin, J. C. (2014). Chronic low-grade inflammation in metabolic disorders: relevance for behavioral symptoms. *NeuroImmunoModulation, 21(2–3)*, 95 - 101.

Pereira, S. A.-L. (2014). Low-grade inflammation, obesity, and diabetes. *Curr. Obes. Rep., 3(4)*, 422 - 431.

Sclomet, D. L.-H. (2018). Revisiting the carrageenan controversy: Do we really understand the digestive fate and safety of carrageenan in our foods? *Royal Society of Chemistry: Food & Function,* 14 - 16.

Thixton, S. (2015). *Why carrageenan can be dangerous to your pet.* Retrieved from Pet Food Safety Advocate: Truth about pet food.com: https://truthaboutpetfood.com/why-carrageenan-can-be-dangerous-to-your-pet/

WebMD. (2019). *Carrageenan.* Retrieved from WebMD: https://www.webmd.com/vitamins/ai/ingredientmono-710/carrageenan

WHO. (2015). *Safety and evaluation of certain food additives.* Geneva: WHO: Prepared by the 79th meeting joint FAO / WHO expert committee on food additives.

Guar Gum

Alternate names, (a.k.a.): Gellan gum, hydroxypropyl guar, guaran, galactomannan polysaccharide, guar bean extract

Purpose: Used as a filler to increase bulk and as a thickening agent; Because it is gluten-free, it is used as an additive to replace wheat flour in baked goods. Guar gum is a thickening agent in foods and medicines for humans and animals.

Guar gum, when used as a food additive, also has *functional food* qualities in it that its high-fiber content may minimally help lower cholesterol and glycemic index (Brown, 1999).

Found in many processed foods, including salad dressings, soups, baked goods, beverages, cream cheese, ricotta cheese, ice cream, and other frozen desserts. In medications, it is a water-soluble fiber that acts as a bulk-forming laxative and promotes regular now movements.

ADI: None

Maximum Daily Intake (MDI): The FDA has specific maximum usage levels for different types of food products, ranging from 0.35% in baked goods to 2% in processed vegetable juices (FDA, 2018). For example, coconut milk has a maximum guar gum usage level of 1%. Therefore, 1-cup (240-gram) serving can contain a maximum of 2.4 grams of guar gum (Link, 2017). Consuming too many foods or too many portions of food containing guar gum can cause adverse side effects.

Additional Information
Guar gum is an indigestible polysaccharide, an insoluble fiber, which is good for our digestion and large-intestine microbiota. Guar gum requires a large amount of water to pass through the intestines. If a body is dehydrated or does not drink enough water, it will absorb as much water as needed from our intestines, which can cause dehydration or bowel obstruction (FDA, 1991).

Guar gum is also capable of reducing the absorbability of dietary minerals. Soy protein occurs as an impurity in manufactured guar gum and can make up as much as 10%. The guar gum can, therefore, adversely affect those with sensitivity to soy (Marks, 2017).

Side effects

Allergic reaction/ Anaphylaxis	Irritable bowel symptoms
Bloating	Nasal congestion/ Runny nose
Chest Pain; Tightness	Shortness of breath
Constipation	Skin rashes
Coughing	Sores and lesions along inside intestines
Diarrhea	Soy proteins allergy
Esophageal blockage	Vomiting / Nausea
Hives	Watery eyes / Itchy eyes
Intestinal blockage	Wheezing

People who experience any of the above symptoms or take medication for them may want to avoid foods and medications containing guar gum. Anyone with the following conditions should also avoid guar gum:

- ✓ Intestinal obstructions
- ✓ Swallowing food
- ✓ Irritable bowel symptoms
- ✓ Soy allergies

References

Brown, L. R. (1999). Cholesterol-lowering effects of dietary fiber: a meta-analysis. *The American Journal of Clinical Nutrition, 69(1)*, 30-42.

FDA. (1991). Supplements: Making sure hype does not overwhelm science . *Food and Drug Administration.*

FDA. (2018). *Sec. 184.1339 Guar gum.* Retrieved from TITLE 21--FOOD AND DRUG Administration: Human Health Services: https://www.accessdata.fda.gov/scripts/cdrh/cfdocs/cfcfr/CFRSearch.cfm?fr= 184.1339

Link, R. (2017). *Is guar gum healthy or unhealthy?* Retrieved from Healthline: https://www.healthline.com/nutrition/guar-gum

Marks, D. (2017). *Guar gum.* Retrieved from Healthfully: https://healthfully.com/316045-guar-gum-and-soy-allergy.html

High Fructose Corn Syrup

Alternate names (a.k.a.): Fructose, Corn syrup, Isoglucose, Maize syrup, Glucose syrup, Fruit fructose, Crystalline fructose, fruit sugar, HFCS

Found in many processed foods, beverages, and medications in the USA. It is a thick liquid found in most yogurts, ketchup, cereals, pancake syrup, ice-cream, soft drinks, cookies, canned soup, fruit juices, candy, cookies, desserts, cake mixes, canned vegetables, bread, and most other processed food items.

Purpose: HFCS enhances flavor. It blends more easily into beverages than table sugar and has great preservative qualities that are used in processed foods to extend their shelf life.

Nutritional Value: None; our body does not require added sugar and does not process HFCS the same way our body processes other organic sugars

ADI: "The American Heart Association (AHA) recommends no more than 6 teaspoons (25 grams) of added sugar per day for women and 9 teaspoons (38 grams) for men, (Johnson, 2009) The AHA limits for children vary depending on their age and caloric needs, but range between 3-6 teaspoons (12 - 25 grams) per day" (UCSF Sugar Science, n.d.).

The World Health Organization's (WHO) recommendation that no more than 10% of an adult's calories and ideally less than 5% should come from added sugar or from natural sugars in honey, syrups, and fruit juice. For a 2,000-calorie diet, 5% would be 25 grams

Derived from corn: GMO corn and Maize.

Additional Information:

"The levels of all sugars consumed per person in the U.S. has increased from 4 pounds a year in 1776 to 20 pounds in 1850, to 120 pounds in 1994, and now 160 pounds per person per year. Much of this increase in sugar consumption is from HFCS, especially in the form of soft drinks and processed foods" (Sharon, 2018).

High fructose corn syrup does not exist in nature. HFCS is genetically modified. When this artificial sweetener was introduced into the American food supply, children for the first time began getting type II diabetes, and obesity rates soared. In at least one study, the syrup has been linked to both.

Research shows that HFCS interferes with people's metabolism in such a way as to make people feel hungrier than they really are. This is because HFCS decreases the secretion of leptin into the body's system and increases the production of ghrelin, which sends your appetite into over-drive.

The human body does not have enzymes capable of digesting HFCS; instead, HFCS is metabolized by the liver. The pancreas cannot release insulin the way it normally does for sugar, so fructose is converted to fat and stored.

Also, some research has found low levels of mercury in HFCS due to how it is processed. Given the high volume of HFCS in the American diet, this could be a significant source of mercury exposure, which should be further researched (Highfructosecornsyrup.org, 2009).

"90 percent of America's corn and soybeans are genetically modified, and producers of eggs, milk, and meat rely on those crops to feed their animals. Soy oil and corn starch are used throughout the industry" (Charles, 2013).

"HFCS is derived from corn starch. Starch itself is a chain of glucose (a simple sugar) molecules joined together. When corn starch is broken down into individual glucose molecules, the end product is corn syrup, which is essentially 100% glucose. To make HFCS, enzymes are added to corn syrup in order to convert some of the glucose into a simple sugar called fructose, because it occurs naturally in fruits and berries. HFCS is 'high' in fructose compared to the pure glucose that is in corn syrup. Different formulations of HFCS contain different amounts of fructose" (FDA, 2019)

"Research shows that high-fructose corn syrup changes animal metabolism and is actually metabolized much differently than other sugars. HFCS is a highly processed product that contains nearly the same amount of fructose and glucose. High-fructose corn syrup metabolizes into fat in your body much faster than other sugars, resulting in increased fat gain" (Barrett, 2012).

Organic sugars, in their natural form, pass through the digestive tract. Most unused energy from these sugars is excreted from the body, whereas concentrated high fructose corn syrup processed by the liver, where it is then converted to fat and stored in the abdomen in the form of triglycerides. This increases your blood levels of triglycerides and increases your risk for heart disease, diabetes, or both put together make metabolic syndrome (Rippe, 2013).

Every cell in your body, including your brain, utilizes glucose. Therefore, much of it is "burned up" immediately after you consume it. By contrast, fructose is turned into free fatty acids and triglycerides, which get stored as fat. The fatty acids created during fructose metabolism accumulate as fat droplets in your liver and skeletal muscle tissues, causing insulin resistance and non-alcoholic fatty liver disease. Insulin resistance progresses to metabolic syndrome and type II diabetes. In other words, fructose converts to fat, which is directly turned into triglycerides.

Glucose does not do this. When you eat 120 calories of glucose, less than one calorie is stored as fat compared to 120 calories of fructose results in 40 calories stored as fat. Glucose suppresses your hunger hormone ghrelin and stimulates leptin to suppress your appetite, but HFCS interferes with your brain's communication with leptin, resulting in overeating (Mercola, 2013).

Typically, food labels list ingredients in the order of which is the most to least. Dieticians recommend not consuming any processed foods that list any form of sugar in its first three ingredients, because it means that produce is mostly sugar. How some sneaky processed food producers fool and get around this simple rule is by using many different names listed individually. For example, ketchup, cookies, or other products may list HFCS, corn syrup, corn starch, and isoglucose syrup as the fourth, fifth, ninth, and tenth ingredients. All breakdown to the same molecules by the liver that converts it to triglyceride fat stored in the belly.

"Fructose in Fruit vs. Fructose in High Fructose Corn Syrup: Studies have shown that the natural sugar fructose in fruit is metabolized in the body differently than the fructose in HFCS. The absorption of natural fructose in fruit is slowed down and buffered by the fiber, antioxidants, and phytonutrients contained in the fruit. As such, the spike in blood sugar, the corresponding rise in blood insulin levels, and then subsequent rebound dip into hypoglycemia observed after consumption of HFCS is not observed in the consumption of fruit. In fact, studies have shown that even daily consumption of 20 servings of fruit a day does not negatively impact blood sugar levels" (Sharon, 2018).

Current results of the research provide evidence that sugar consumption at the level of 25% of total caloric intake increases risk factors for cardiovascular disease. HFCS increases fasting LDL cholesterol and triglycerides. It also causes a quick high glucose level with a rapid drop after eating. These results contradict the previous Dietary Guidelines for Americans, which recommended a maximal upper limit of 25% of total energy requirements from added sugar. Current research indicated this number might need to be reevaluated and greatly reduced (Kimber L. Stanhope, 2011).

High fructose corn syrup has been found to contain trace amounts of mercury as a result of some manufacturing processes. Its consumption can lead to zinc loss. Amongst other dietary factors, learning and behavior are influenced not only by nutrients but also by exposure to toxic food contaminants that can disrupt metabolic processes and cause neurological-developmental disorders such as autism, mental retardation, and attention deficit hyperactivity disorder. These dietary factors may be directly related to the development of behavior disorders and learning disabilities. Since high fructose corn syrup is a common ingredient in many processed foods and beverages, it's consumption should be considered in those individuals with nutritional deficits such as zinc deficiency or who are allergic or sensitive to the effects of mercury or unable to effectively metabolize and eliminate it from the body, (Dufault, 2009).

Moderate and frequent consumption of HFCS, including fruit juices that are made with 100% fruit juice, increased asthma risk, independent of age, sex, smoking, BMI. This may be because of the high fructose malabsorption and formation of asthma-triggering immunogens in the digestive system. Recommendations are to reduce sugar-sweetened beverages and 100 % juice (DeChristopher, 2018).

Banned in Other Countries: Yes

Side Effects

Asthma	Insulin resistance
Attention Deficit Hyperactivity Disorder	Indigestion
Autism	Intestinal tumors, cancer
Behavioral problems	Learning Disabilities
Breathing Problems / Shortness of breath	Leptin resistance

Chest Pain, tightness, fluttering, pressure	Liver failure; fatty liver
Confusion, forgetfulness, dementia	Metabolic syndrome
Diabetes	Neurological disabilities
High Cholesterol	Obesity

People who experience any of the above symptoms or take medication for them may want to avoid foods and medications containing HFCS. Anyone with the following conditions should also avoid HFCS:

✓ Asthma
✓ Attention Deficit Hyperactivity Disorder (ADHD)
✓ Behavioral problems: Moodiness, anger, violent tendencies
✓ Diabetes
✓ Cancer
✓ Cholesterol: High LDL or Triglycerides
✓ Memory loss
✓ Metabolic syndrome: Heart disease + Diabetes
✓ Neurological disorders: Parkinson's, multiple sclerosis
✓ Obesity
✓ Respiratory Distress / Shortness of Breath
✓ Pregnant

Reference

Barrett, M. (2012). *Human Metabolism Negatively Impacted by High-Fructose Corn Syrup*. Retrieved from Natural Society: https://naturalsociety.com/high-fructose-corn-syrup-alters-human-metabolism/

Charles, D. (2013). *How American food companies Go GMO-free In a GMO world*. Retrieved from NPR: https://www.npr.org/sections/thesalt/2014/02/04/269479079/how-american-food-companies-go-gmo-free-in-a-gmo-world

DeChristopher, L. T. (2018). Excess free fructose, high-fructose corn syrup, and adult asthma: the Framingham Offspring Cohort. *British Journal of Nutrition*, 1157-1167.

Dufault, R. S. (2009). Mercury exposure, nutritional deficiencies, and metabolic disruptions may affect learning in children. *Behavioral Brain Function, 5-44.*

FDA. (2019). *High Fructose Corn Syrup: Q & A's*. Retrieved from Food and Drug Administration: https://www.fda.gov/food/food-additives-petitions/high-fructose-corn-syrup-questions-and-answers

Highfructosecornsyrup.org. (2009). *Guess what's lurking in your food*. Retrieved from Highfructosecornsyrup.org: http://www.highfructosecornsyrup.org/2009/02/guess-whats-lurking-in-your-food.html

Johnson, R. A.-R. (2009). *Dietary Sugars Intake and Cardiovascular Health A Scientific Statement From the American Heart Association*. Retrieved from AHA Journals;DOI: 10.1161/CIRCULATIONAHA.109.192627, p. 1011 - 1020.: https://www.ahajournals.org/doi/pdf/10.1161/circulationaha.109.192627

Kimber L. Stanhope, A. A. (2011). Consumption of fructose and high fructose corn syrup increase postprandial triglycerides, LDL-cholesterol, and apolipoprotein-B in young men and women. *Journal of Endocrinology Metabolism, 96(10)*, EJournal of Endocrinology Metabolism. Retrieved from Journal of Endocrinology Metabolism.

Mercola, J. (2013). *Fructose can increase hunger and lead to overeating*. Retrieved from Dr. Mercola: https://articles.mercola.com/sites/articles/archive/2013/01/14/fructose-spurs-overeating.aspx#_edn6

Rippe, J. A. (2013). Sucrose, High-Fructose Corn Syrup, and fructose, their metabolism, and potential health effects: What do we really know? *Advances in Nutrition 4(2)l Oxford Academy*, 236-245.

Sharon. (2018). *High Fructose Corn Syrup*. Retrieved from Nutritionfacts.org: https://nutritionfacts.org/topics/high-fructose-corn-syrup/

UCSF Sugar Science. (n.d.). *How much is too much?* Retrieved from Sugar Science; University of San Francisco: https://sugarscience.ucsf.edu/the-growing-concern-of-overconsumption.html#.XPa5l3dFyH8

Mono Sodium Gluconate

Alternate names, a.k.a.: MSG, sodium gluconate, Ajinomoto, calcium gluconate, iron gluconate, magnesium gluconate, potassium gluconate, zinc gluconate, glutamic acid

Ingredients that may contain MSG:

Autolyzed yeast	Hydrolyzed protein
Calcium caseinate	Monopotassium glutamate
Gelatin	Sodium caseinate
Glutamate	Textured protein

"MSG and related toxins are often added to foods in disguised forms. For example, among the food manufacturers, favorite disguises are 'hydrolyzed vegetable protein,' 'vegetable protein,' 'natural flavorings,' and 'spices.' Each of these may contain from 12 percent to 40 percent MSG" (American Nutrition Association, 2019).

As required by the FDA, monosodium glutamate is listed on the label of any food to which it is added. However, other chemically distinct glutamate additives may, in some sensitive individuals, induce similar symptoms. They include (Healthpedian.org, 2019):

- Autolyzed yeast
- Calcium caseinate
- Hydrolyzed protein
- Maltodextrin
- Modified food starch
- Monopotassium glutamate
- Sodium caseinate
- Textured protein

Purpose: Enhance flavor, tenderize meat, preserve food. It is used in some medications to improve potassium as an electrolyte and improve mineral absorption.

Found in many processed foods, everything from canned to frozen foods; and everything from candy, soda, and other desserts to meat, dairy, soups, chips, and vegetable products.

Nutritional Value: None

Daily recommended Amount: The FDA recommends no more than 2,300 milligrams of sodium per day in healthy individuals. Certain groups should limit intake to 1,500 milligrams per day:

- Children
- Over the age of 50
- Anyone with diabetes, heart disease or kidney disease

FDA: GRAS

Additional Information

"The science supporting the relationship between sodium reduction and health is clear: When sodium intake increases, blood pressure increases, and high blood pressure is a major risk factor for heart disease and stroke – two leading causes of death in the U.S. The CDC compiled a number of key studies, which continue to support the benefits of sodium reduction in lowering blood pressure. Researchers estimate the lowering of U.S. sodium intake by about 40 percent over the next decade could save 500,000 lives and nearly $100 billion in healthcare costs" (FDA, 2011).

"The majority of sodium consumed comes from processed and prepared foods, not the saltshaker. This makes it difficult for all of us to control how much sodium we consume" (FDA, 2011).

"A recent study supports that elevated dietary MSG consumption is significantly associated with having metabolic syndrome and being overweight. A person with daily consumption of MSG exceeding 5 g should be considered at risk for metabolic disorder" (Insawang, 2012).

"A possible role for nitric oxide in glutamate (MSG)-induced Chinese restaurant syndrome, glutamate-induced asthma, 'hot-dog headache,' pugilistic Alzheimer's disease, and other disorders," (Scher, 1992).

"MSG has been used as a food additive for decades. Over the years, the FDA has received many anecdotal reports of adverse reactions to foods containing MSG. These reactions are known as MSG symptoms. However, researchers have found no definitive evidence of a link between MSG and these symptoms. Researchers acknowledge, though, that a small percentage of people may have short-term reactions to MSG. Symptoms are usually mild and don't require treatment. The only way to prevent a reaction is to avoid foods containing MSG" (Drugs.com, 2018).

Many biochemicals can act as neurotransmitters in the brain. These are known as excitotoxins because they excite our neurons (nerves). MSG excites our neurons. Additives that may contain MSG and/or other excitotoxins: Soy Protein Concentrate; Soy Protein Isolate Whey; Protein Concentrate, (American Nutrition Association, 2019).

Research shows that people who suffer from allergies or severe asthma may be susceptible to MSG sensitivity. Some studies have also found that patients with asthma may have more severe asthma attacks after ingesting MSG. MSG intolerance is not considered an allergy because it does not involve a reaction by the immune system. As with all food sensitivities, the best way to treat MSG sensitivity (or intolerance) is to avoid MSG" (Healthpedian.org, 2019).

Effects

Allergic reactions/ Asthmatic attack	Hyperactivity
Angina / Chest pain	Increase hunger/appetite
Bloating	Insomnia
Breathing difficulty	Insulin resistance
Burning/ numbness in the back of the neck	Joint pain
Burning/numbness in the mouth	Kidney disease
Confusion/ cloudy thinking	Leptin resistance
Degenerative disc or bone disease	Mental confusion
Degenerative muscle disease	Memory Impairment
Depression	Nausea
Diabetes	Neurological disorders
Diarrhea	Obesity
Drowsiness/ fatigue	Rapid heart rate / fluttering
Facial tightness or pressure	Runny nose / congestion
Flushing	Seizures
Headaches / migraines	Shortness of breath
Heart palpitations	Stroke
Heartburn	Sweating
High blood pressure	Tingling, warmth sensations
Hives	Vascular disease / circulation problems
Hot flashes	♣ Weakness

♣   Anything that may cause muscle weakness applies to all muscle strength, including those in our organs and body tissues. Muscle weakness can affect your body's ability to digest food, your lung's ability to breath, or your heart's ability to pump blood.

Who should avoid MSG: Anyone experiencing or taking medication for side effects listed above. Anyone with the following conditions:
- ✓ Anxiety disorders
- ✓ Diabetes
- ✓ Degenerative diseases: Degenerative disc disease, herniated discs, osteomyelitis
- ✓ Fibromyalgia
- ✓ Headache

- ✓ Heart disease
- ✓ Kidney disease or failure
- ✓ Learning disabilities
- ✓ Memory loss, dementia, Alzheimer's
- ✓ Mental disorders
- ✓ Metabolic syndrome =Diabetes + Heart disease
- ✓ Neurologic diseases: Parkinson's, Multiple Sclerosis, Gillian Barrett, Amyotrophic Lateral Sclerosis (ALS, Lou Gehrig's disease)
- ✓ Obesity
- ✓ Pregnancy: Fetus' exposed to excitotoxins may cause neurological disorders

Rebekah S. Mead

References

American Nutrition Association. (2019). *Review of :Excitotoxinsl the taste that kills.* Retrieved from American Nutrition Association; Nutrition Digest, 38(2): http://americannutritionassociation.org/newsletter/review-excitotoxins-taste-kills

Drugs.com. (2018). *Monosodium Glutamate.* Retrieved from Drugs.com: https://www.drugs.com/mcf/monosodium-glutamate-msg-is-it-harmful

FDA. (2011). *Sodium Reduction.* Retrieved from Food and Drug Administration: https://www.fda.gov/food/food-additives-petitions/sodium-reduction

Healthpedian.org. (2019). *MSG sensitivity (Intolerance): causes, symptoms, and treatment.* Retrieved from Healthopedia.com: https://www.healthpedian.org/msg-sensitivity-intolerance-causes-symptoms-and-treatment/

Insawang, T. S. (2012). Monosodium glutamate (MSG) intake is associated with the prevalence of metabolic syndrome in a rural Thai population. *Nutri Metabolism, 9 (50).*

Scher, W. S. (1992). A possible role for nitric oxide in glutamate (MSG)-induced Chinese restaurant syndrome, glutamate-induced asthma, 'hot-dog headache,' pugilistic Alzheimer's disease, and other disorders. *Medical Hypothesis, 38(3),* 185-188.

Phosphoric Acid

Alternate names, a.k.a): Orthophosphoric acid, Hydrogen phosphate, E338, Phosphoric(V) acid, Pyrophosphoric acid, Triphosphoic acid, o-Phosphoric acid

Purpose: Gives beverages and foods a tangy acidic flavor. It inhibits bacteria and mold growth in sugary foods. It helps to regulate acidity and used to enhance the flavor of poultry and meat products.

Found in: Cola beverages, bottled and canned iced teas, bottled and canned coffee beverages, breakfast cereal bars, nondairy creamers, and processed cheeses; used to enhance the flavor of older cuts of chicken and meat products. The salts of phosphoric acid are used in many dairy products to modify the proteins and alter the pH to produce a higher-quality product — the addition of phosphates derived from phosphoric acid to cheese results in smooth, shelf-stable products. Phosphoric acid and phosphate food additives are added to milk, buttermilk, cottage cheese, and nondairy coffee creamers. It is also in many pet foods.

ADI: None; not recommended for children or teens because it can affect bone development.

Nutritional value: None

FDA: GRAS

Additional Information

Phosphorus binds more readily to the same receptor sites in bones as calcium; therefore, it weakens bone strength and makes your body more susceptible to bone fractures.

Food grade phosphoric acid toxicology reports indicate this is a corrosive and warns of potential harm to target organs, blood, liver, and bone marrow (CCI, 2018).

Due to its high acidity level, phosphoric acid can erode tooth enamel and make your teeth more prone to decay. The addition of phosphoric acid and sugar in most soda dramatically increases the risk of tooth decay (Shidara, 2014).

Phosphoric acid also has the potential to contribute to the formation of kidney stones, especially in those who have had kidney stones previously (Qaseem, 2014).

"Cola intake was associated with significantly lower Bone Mineral Density (BMD) at each hip site, but not the spine, in women but not in men. The mean BMD of those with daily cola intake was 3.7% lower at the femoral neck and 5.4% lower at Ward's area than of those who consumed more than one serving of cola per month. The calcium-to-phosphorus ratios were lower" (Tucker KL, 2006).

"Among physically active girls, the cola beverages, in particular, are highly associated with bone fractures" (Wyshak, 2000).

"Carbonated beverage consumption has been linked with diabetes, hypertension, and kidney stones, all risk factors for chronic kidney disease. Cola beverages, in particular, contain phosphoric acid and have been associated with urinary changes that promote kidney stones. Drinking 2 or more servings per of cola per day was associated with increased risk of chronic kidney disease" (Saldana, 2007).

"Excess phosphorus in your diet can decrease your body's calcium levels. Also, it can lead to phosphorus overload, which can impair your body's utilization of vital nutrients like iron, magnesium, and zinc" (Price, 2017).

Consuming an excess amount of phosphorus in your diet can decrease your body's calcium levels resulting in reduced bone density. Research links daily consumption to hypocalcemia. Also, it can lead to phosphorus overload, which can impair your body's utilization of vital nutrients like iron, magnesium, and zinc. Deficiencies in any of these nutrients can lead to all kinds of other health problems (Price, 2019).

Physically active teenaged girls who drink a lot of beverages high in phosphoric acid have a high incidence of bone fractures. The results of this research confirm that previous findings are associating bone fractures in physically active girls with carbonated beverages high in phosphoric acid. The results have policy implications for improving the dietary practices and health of children (Wyshak, 2000)

Consumption of food and beverages high in phosphoric acid can lead to chronic kidney stones (Saldana T. B., 2007).

Banned in other countries: Unknown

Side Effects:

Bone Fractures in teens	Microbiota, changes
Dermatitis	Muscle pain, weakness
Diarrhea	Pain, chronic, fibromyalgia
Hip fractures, spontaneous in elderly	Stomach cramps
Immune deficiency	Stomach acid imbalance
Iron deficiency	Tooth decay & mitral valve disease
Kidney stones	Zinc deficiency
Magnesium deficiency	Osteoporosis/ loss of bone density

Anyone taking medications for any of the above symptoms or have the following conditions may want to avoid food and medications that contain this ingredient:
- ✓ Children and teenagers
- ✓ Degenerative disorders: Osteoporosis, degenerative disc disease, weak muscles
- ✓ Hip fractures
- ✓ Kidney stones

References

CCI. (2018). *Safety Data Sheet: phosphoric acid 20% w/w food grade.* Columbia, WI: Columbus Chemical Industries.

Price, A. (2017). *Phosphoric acid: The dangerous hidden additive you've likely consumed.* Retrieved from Dr. Axe: https://draxe.com/phosphoric-acid/

Qaseem, A. D. (2014). Dietary and pharmacologic management to prevent recurrent nephrolithiasis in adults: A clinical practice guideline from the American College of Physicians". *Annals of Internal Medicine, 161, 9,* 659-667.

Saldana, T. B. (2007). Carbonated beverage. *Epidemiology, 18(4),* 501-506.

Shidara, C. (2014). *Diet Soda, Fruit Juices are Also Bad for Your Teeth.* Retrieved from Contra Costa Health Services: https://cchealth.org/column/2014-0228-healthy-outlook.php

Tucker KL, M. K. (2006). Colas, but not other carbonated beverages, are associated with low bone mineral density in older women: The Framingham Osteoporosis Study. *American Journal of Clinical Nutrition, 84(4),* 936-942.

Wyshak, G. (2000). Teenaged Girls, Carbonated Beverage Consumption, and Bone Fractures. *Pediatric Adolescent Medicine, 154(6),* 610-613.

Potassium Bromate

Alternate Names (a.k.a.): Potassium bromate, bromate, bromated flour, bromated vegetable oil

Purpose: A synthetic reagent, oxidizer, and food additive. Used in strengthen and add elasticity to processed flours that have most or all of its gluten (grain protein) removed.

Bromate is used to treat malt barley during the production of beer and other consumable products (Ministry of Health and Welfare, Japan, 1979). Many fast-food restaurants serve bagels, bread pizza dough, and buns made with potassium bromate.

Potassium Bromate can be found in (Farrow, 2013):

- Pesticides (methyl bromide),
- Bread products: Pizza crust, bread, bagels, chips, crackers
- Brominated vegetable oil added to citrus-flavored drinks
- Disinfectant cleansers
- Asthma inhalers
- Prescription drugs
- Cosmetics
- plastic products, some personal care products

Additional Information:

"Potassium bromate is an oxidizing agent used to strengthens dough to allow higher rising. Under the right conditions, it is safe in baking bread. However, if too much is added, or if the bread is not baked long enough or not at a high enough temperature, then a residual amount may remain, which may be harmful if consumed (Kurokawa, 1990)" (Wolf, 1998).

"In a final rule for bromate, U.S. EPA (1998a) stated that "there is sufficient laboratory animal data to conclude that bromate is a probable human carcinogen." The U.S. EPA had classified bromate as a Group B2 carcinogen in 1993 (U.S. EPA, 1993). This finding was also identified in a 1998 Health Risk Assessment (U.S. EPA, 1998b), which concluded: "bromate should be evaluated as a likely human carcinogen by the oral route of exposure."

"In all of the cited case studies, when bromate was administered as potassium bromate, the potassium bromate was listed as causing cancer under Proposition 65 on January 1, 1990. Potassium bromate is readily soluble in water. Thus, U.S. EPA refers to a dose of bromate in its documents and characterizes the potential for carcinogenicity following bromate exposure (U.S. EPA, 1993; 1998a; b)" (California EPA, 2001).

"A higher protein baking flour that does not contain potassium bromate is most desirable. The higher protein allows the flour to develop more gluten, which results in a more stable baked product and also is desirable for bakers in high altitudes. Potassium bromate is typically added to bread flour to help the elasticity of the baked product. The additive is not permitted for use in the U.K., but it is used in the U.S. Many consider potassium bromate unhealthful, and products that contain the additive must be labeled as such in the U.S.," (Gourmet Sleuth, n.d.).

"Banned from use in food products in Europe and Canada. It has not been banned in the United States, but the U.S. Food and Drug Administration asked bakers to choose other additives voluntarily, and federal regulations limit the amount that can be added to flour. Following guidelines established under its Safe Drinking Water and Toxic Enforcement Act, the State of California includes potassium bromate on its list of chemicals known to cause cancer and requires products containing bromated flour to carry a warning label," (Busch, 2017).

"These results show that potassium bromates ($KBrO_3$) have seriously damaging effects on the central nervous system, and therefore, its use should be avoided (Ajarem, 2016).

"Potassium bromate can disrupt the genetic material within cells. (EPA, 2001). Upon entering the body, potassium bromate can be transformed into molecules called oxides and radicals. These highly reactive molecules can damage DNA and may play a role in the development of cancer. Scientists have observed such damage in human liver and intestine cells, where exposure to potassium bromate resulted in breaks in DNA strands and chromosomal damage, (Zhang Y, 2011). Researchers also saw significant damage to the cell membranes of the small intracellular bodies responsible for important cell functions such as cellular digestion, ironically, the process by which food is broken down into components useful to our cells. Models of the relationship between DNA damage and potassium bromate show a consistent low-dose linear response, which means that the amount of DNA damage observed is proportional to the amount of potassium bromate consumed (Spassova, 2019)." (EWG, 2015)

Potassium Bromate can be rapidly absorbed into the intestines and cause nausea, diarrhea, vomiting, stomach pains, muscle weakness, hearing loss, kidney failure. (EPA, 2001).

In 2007 the India Times reported that China removed entire batches of chips produced in the USA because they contained Potassium Bromate, which its use was banned for many years before that (Neelakantan, 2016).

"No epidemiological studies available. Data collected is from reports in humans following accidental or suicidal ingestion of permanent hair wave neutralizing solution. These products usually contain either 2% potassium bromate, or 10% sodium bromate. The most common acute signs are severe gastrointestinal irritation, central nervous system (CNS) depression, renal failure, and hearing loss" (EPA, 2001).

New Jersey Department of Health and Senior Services & Environmental Protection Agency (NJDEP, 2005). Hazard Summary:

- Used as a lab reagent and an oxidizer when used as a food additive

- Carcinogenic: Use with extreme caution

- Breathed in can cause nose, throat and lung irritation including wheezing and shortness of breath

- Contact with skin can cause burns

- Repeated exposure can cause problems with the nervous system: Headaches, irritability, impaired thinking and personality changes

- May cause damage to kidneys

Banned in one or more other Countries: Yes

Side Effect (Kurowawa, 1990) (Entezam, 2010) (EPA, 2001) (NJDEP, 2005) and the above resources:

Anxiety

Cancer: Heart, lungs, kidneys

Cancer: Skin

Cancer: Mesothelioma

Depression

Dizziness

DNA lesions

Ear nerve damage/ Hearing loss

Ear nerve damage/ Balance problems

Headaches/migraines

Impaired digestion

Impaired thinking; confusion

Irritability

Kidney failure

Muscle weakness

Nerve damage; General

Stomach pains

People who experience any of the above symptoms or take medication for them may want to avoid foods and medications containing this ingredient. Also, anyone with the following conditions may want to avoid foods containing this ingredient:

- ✓ Balance problems, clumsiness
- ✓ Mesothelioma cancer that starts with the lining of lungs, heart, kidneys, digestive system
- ✓ Renal/Kidney Tumors & Cancer
- ✓ Adrenal Tumors & Cancer
- ✓ Thyroid Tumors & Cancer
- ✓ Perineum (the area between anus and scrotum or vagina) Cancer
- ✓ Pericardium (lining around the heart) Cancer
- ✓ Skin cancer
- ✓ Inner ear disturbances
- ✓ Neurologic disorders

References

Ajarem, J. A.-M. (2016). Oral administration of potassium bromate induces neurobehavioral changes, alters cerebral neurotransmitters level, and impairs brain tissue of swiss mice — b*ehavioral Brain Function, 12*, 14.

Busch, S. (2017). *Long-term health impact of bromated flour.* Retrieved from Healthfully.com: https://healthfully.com/549792-long-term-health-impact-of-bromated-flour.html

California EPA. (2001). *Reproductive and Cancer Hazard Assessment Section: Potassium Bromate.* Retrieved from Chemical meeting the criteria for listing as cancer-causing via the authoratative body mechanisms; PACKAGE 19a.1.a California EPA: https://oehha.ca.gov/media/downloads/proposition-65/chemicals/noilabpkg19a1a.pdf

EPA. (2001). *Toxicology review of bromate.* Washington, D.C.: U.S. Environmental Protection Agency.

EPA. (2001). *Toxicology review of bromate (CAS No. 15541-45-4).* Washington, D.C.: Environmental Protection Agency.

EWG. (2015). *Potassium Bromate.* Retrieved from EWG.org: https://www.ewg.org/research/potassium-bromate

Farrow, L. (2013). *The iodine crisis.* Devon Press.

Gourmet Sleuth. (n.d.). *What is unbromated flour?* Retrieved from The Gourmet Sleuth: https://www.gourmetsleuth.com/ingredients/detail/unbromated-flour

Kurokawa, Y. M. (1990). Toxicity and carcinogenicity of potassium bromate--a new renal carcinogen. *Environmental Health Perspective*, 309 - 335.

Ministry of Health and Welfare, Japan. (1979). *Potassium Bromate: The Japanese standards of.* Japan: Ministry of Health and Welfare, (4) p. 367. Retrieved from Inchem.org: http://www.inchem.org/documents/jecfa/jecmono/v18je13.htm

Spassova, M. M. (2019). *Dose-response analysis of bromate-induced DNA damage and mutagenicity is consistent with low-dose linear, no threshold processes.* Lincoln, NE: University of Nebraska EPA.

Wolf, D. C. (1998). Time- and Dose-Dependent Development of Potassium Bromate-Induced Tumors in Male Fischer 344 Rats*&da. *Toxicologic Pathology, 26 (6)*, 724-729.

Zhang, Y, J. L. (2011). Possible involvement of oxidative stress in potassium bromate-induced genotoxicity in Human HepG2 cells. *Chem Biol Interact. 189(3): 186-91.*, 186 - 191.

GMO Soy
Soy Additives & Textured Soy Protein Products

Alternate names, a.k.a.: Hydrolyzed soy protein, HSP, textured vegetable protein, TVP, lecithin, soy sauce, bean sprouts.

Ingredients made from soy: Monosodium Glutamate (MSG), mono-glycerides, diglycerides, teriyaki sauce, bean sprouts, edamame (fresh soybeans), kinako, miso (fermented soybean paste), natto (fermented soybeans with beneficial bacteria), okara, shoyu (a natural soy sauce), soya, soybean curds and granules, tamari, tempeh, tofu, yuba

Other ingredients may or may not contain soy. It is essential to contact the manufacturer of the product to find out the source of the ingredient if trying to avoid organic or GMO soy. These include (Castle, 2019):

Bulking agents	Mixed tocopherols
Hydrolyzed plant protein (HPP)	Natural flavoring
Hydrolyzed vegetable protein (HVP)	Stabilizer
Gum Arabic	Thickener
Guar gum	Vegetable gum, starch, shortening, or oil
Lecithin	Vitamin E

Purpose: Flavorings, preservatives, sweeteners, emulsifiers, thickeners, and used to make synthetic nutrients, imitation seafood, meat, butter, cheese, milk, and eggs. It is also used in medications.

Found in: Almost every processed food. It is used to imitate many organic foods, such as seafood, hamburgers, hotdogs, and sausage.

ADI: See section on recommendations for protein and fat intake

Nutritional Value: High in protein and low in saturated fat

Additional Information

Soybeans sold in the USA can be organic, non-GMO, or GMO glyphosate & dicamba-tolerant.

In America, 94% of all soy produced and sold in America has been genetically altered. It is found in almost every processed food, including condiments. It is used to mimic many organic foods, including meat, seafood, peanut butter, butter, salad dressing, milk, cheese.

I recently considered buying butter that stated on the front label, "with olive oil," Thinking it may be a healthy choice, I then looked at the ingredients and saw #1 ingredient was canola oil (a GMO oil) and there was also more soy lecithin than cream. The last of eight ingredients were olive oil.

> "In 2018, 94 percent of the soybean crops in the United States were genetically modified to be herbicide-tolerant. By comparison, only 17 percent of soybean crops were genetically modified in 1997" (Statista, 2019).

On another recent shopping expedition, I went to our local fresh fish market to buy some fresh fish. They had stuffed clamshells for $1.50 each. I almost bought a half-dozen when I decided to ask, "does it have any HFCS in it."

The man working the counter said he didn't know but then offered to let me see the package label that was in their freezer.

The ingredient panel listed about fifteen ingredients, of which none were clams or any real foods. I saw six forms of soy, including textured soy (used to mimic clams) and soy lecithin and a bunch of other chemicals that may also come from soy. They were stuffed clamshells, but there were no clams in the stuffing. Instead, they were stuffed with textured vegetable protein (soy), held together with soy oils, and flavored with multiple chemicals, including additional soy additives. The label was deceptive. Those stuffed clamshells did not contain the nutrients typically found in fresh clams, while unsuspecting consumers allergic to soy would be getting a whopping allergic reaction or other side effects.

Since the onset of writing this book, I have since stopped using commercial salad dressings on my organic salads that I mostly grow in my organic garden. I have not been able to find any that do not contain GMO oils, thickeners, and flavor enhancers. I now use just vinegar and oil.

> Soybean contains large quantities of natural toxins or "antinutrients." First among them are potent enzyme inhibitors that block the action of trypsin and other enzymes needed for protein digestion. These inhibitors are large, tightly folded proteins that are not completely

deactivated during ordinary cooking. They can produce severe gastric distress, reduced protein digestion, and chronic deficiencies in amino acid uptake. In test animals, diets high in trypsin inhibitors cause enlargement and disease conditions of the pancreas, including cancer (Mercola, n.d.).

"This evidence report aims to summarize the current evidence on the health effects of soy and its isoflavones on the following: menopausal symptoms, bone health, cancers, cardiovascular diseases, kidney diseases, and cognitive function, as well as safety issues and drug interactions. Also, this report summarizes the formulations of soy products and soy food used in clinical trials. This report is requested and funded by the National Center for Complementary and Alternative Medicine (NCCAM) and the Office of Dietary Supplements at the National Institutes of Health (NIH), through the Evidence-based Practice Center (EPC) program at the Agency for Healthcare Research and Quality" (AHRQ).

October 1999, the U.S. FDA approved a health claim for use on food labels stating that a daily diet containing 25 grams of soy protein is low in saturated fat and cholesterol and may reduce the risk of heart disease. This claim was based on the beneficial results in reducing low-density plasma lipoprotein (LDL) levels from dozens of human-controlled clinical trials. The health claim, however, covers only soy protein, since research results surrounding soy isoflavones were controversial. This report aimed to summarize the formulations of soy products and soy food used in clinical trials, and to reflect the evidence on the health effects, in addition to, safety issues and drug interactions of using soy and its isoflavones as reported in the literature are summarized. "The most frequently reported adverse events were gastrointestinal. These were reported in 33 of 41 comparison studies of soy diets, soy proteins, isoflavones, and phytoestrogen supplements. Menstrual complaints, reported in 15 studies, were also common. Other adverse events included musculoskeletal complaints, headaches, dizziness, and rashes. Also, there were somewhat more withdrawals from the soy arms due to taste aversion" (Balk, 2005).

"Widespread, unpredictable changes: The genetic engineering process creates massive collateral damage, causing mutations in hundreds or thousands of locations throughout the plant's DNA (Latham, 2005). Natural genes can be deleted or permanently turned on or off, and hundreds may change their behavior, (Srivastava, 1999), Even the inserted gene can be damaged or rearranged and may create proteins that can trigger allergies or promote disease.

Genetically modified foods on the market: Almost 98% of Canadian grown canola is genetically engineered for herbicide resistance. U.S. sugar beet production is estimated to be over 95% genetically modified for herbicide resistance. GMO sweet corn, papaya, zucchini, and yellow summer squash are also for sale in grocery stores, but in lesser amounts. Genetically modified alfalfa is grown for use as hay and forage for animals" (IRT, 2019)

Keep in mind that our body needs many nutrients from multiple organic sources; no one grain contains every nutrient needed by our body. Imitation foods cannot provide all the nutrients needed to sustain optimal health.

Banned in other countries: Many countries ban genetically altered soy; some allow milled (ground-up) soy but do not allow it to be cultivated in their country. By grinding / milling it, their GMO seeds cannot accidentally cross-contaminate or be planted and grown in their environment.

Side Effects, (Also see the section on GURT seeds)

Allergies	Kidney, impaired function
Bloating	Learning disabilities
Cholesterol abnormalities	Memory loss
Degenerative bone disease	Menstrual changes in duration

Difficulty swallowing	Menopausal symptoms
Enlarged breasts in males	Moodiness
Heart Disease	Musculoskeletal problems
Headaches	Shortness of breath
Hives	Sluggishness, fatigue
Infertility	Tingling tongue and lips

Anyone taking medications for any of the above symptoms or have the following conditions may want to avoid food and medications that contain this ingredient:

- ✓ Allergic to GMO soy
- ✓ Any form of cancer
- ✓ Breast cancer (see the section on GURT seeds)
- ✓ Crohn's and irritable bowel syndrome
- ✓ Degenerative bone disorders
- ✓ Infertility
- ✓ Kidney disease
- ✓ Menstruation problems

References

Balk, E. C. (2005). *Chapter 126. Effects of Soy on Health Outcomes: Summary.* Rockville, MD: AHRQ.

Castle, J. (2019). *Food choices for a soy-free diet.* Retrieved from Very Well Health.com: https://www.verywellhealth.com/food-and-ingredients-to-avoid-on-a-soy-free-diet-1324000

IRT. (2019). *Health Risks.* Retrieved from Institute for Responsible Technology: https://responsibletechnology.org/gmo-education/health-risks/#5

Latham, J. e. (2005). The Mutational Consequences of Plant Transformation. *The Journal of Biomedicine and Biotechnology.*

Mercola. (n.d.). *Soy health myths debunked.* Retrieved from Dr. Mercola.com: https://www.mercola.com/Downloads/bonus/dangers-of-soy/report.aspx#_edn14

Srivastava, e. a. (1999). Pharmacogenomics of the cystic fibrosis transmembrane conductance regulator (CFTR) and the cystic fibrosis drug CPX using genome microarray analysis. *Molecular Medicine, 11(5),* 753-67.

Statista. (2019). *Percentage of genetically modified crops in the U.S. in 1997 and 2018, by type (as a percent of total acreage).* Retrieved from Statista: https://www.statista.com/statistics/217108/level-of-genetically-modified-crops-in-the-us/

Transglutaminase (Meat Glue)

Alternative names used: TGase, TGN2, TG, TGF, formed meat, reformed meat

Purpose: Transglutaminase is an enzyme found in animals, which helps blood clot, but the food industry can also get it from a type of plant-derived bacteria. Its glue-like properties are used to glue pieces of meat together. It also has thermal stability making it stable as temperature changes, which can help increase the shelf life of dairy products, and it helps thicken dairy products (Romeih, 2017).

"Widely used in various processes: To manufacture cheese and other dairy products, in meat processing, to produce edible films and to manufacture bakery products. Transglutaminase has considerable potential to improve the firmness, viscosity, elasticity, and water-binding capacity of food products" (Kieliszek, 2014).

TG is a naturally occurring enzyme extracted from animals, plants, and bacteria. Most are derived from clotting factors in blood plasma from cows and pigs. Plant-based TG is cultivated using bacteria from vegetable and plant extracts. Most are mixed with other ingredients to create bonds in raw meat strong enough to handle as if they were natural cuts of meat with muscle. It is used primarily by meat producers to reduce waste by gluing small pieces of meat together to form mignon, steaks, roasts, and cuts of meat. TG improves the appearance and texture of formed meats. It can also be used to glue pieces of meat from different animals together, (Arnold, unk.), (Curejoy, 2017), (Gregor M., 2014), (Gregor M., 2015) (P, 2018) (USDA- FSIS, 2001).

Products it is found in (Arnold, Transglutaminase (Meat Glue), n.d.) (Kieliszek, 2014):

- Make steaks out of glued together meat chunks
- Processed meats such as hot dogs, sausage, lunch meats
- Makes imitation crab meat, chicken nuggets, and fish balls
- Creates reconstituted steaks, fillets, roasts, and cutlets
- Makes uniform meat portions that cook evenly and reduce waste

- Binds meat mixtures (sausages, hot dogs) without using casings
- Improves mouth feel, water retention, and appearance of processed meats
- Novel meat combinations like lamb and scallops or bacon and beef.
- Makes meat noodles, shrimp noodles, and other cuisine oddities
- Thickens egg yolks
- Strengthens dough mixtures
- Thickens dairy products (yogurt, cheese)
- Increases yield in tofu production
- Formed cheeses
- Dairy products
- Baked goods
- Cosmetics and skin conditioning products

Daily Allowance: No information found

Additional Information:

"Microbial transglutaminase (mTG) is a food additive, heavily used in a plethora of processed food industries. It is unlabeled and hidden from public knowledge. There are published warnings, alarming the public on the potential danger of using or consuming this enzyme. Recent publications found mTG to be immunogenic in people with celiac disease, and its pathogenicity is continuously unraveled" (Torsten, 2018).

"Meat glue is "used in about eight million pounds of meat every year in the United States, TG has potential food safety and allergy implications" (Gregor, 2014).

Bacterial Contamination from multiple pieces of meat, potentially from different animals, can be a hazard. "When there is a bacteria outbreak, it's much harder to figure out the source" (P, 2018).

According to the USDA-FSIS Tgase ruling in 2001, "Public awareness of all segments of rulemaking and policy development is important. Consequently, to better ensure that minorities, women, and persons with disabilities are aware of this direct final rule, FSIS is responsible for announcing it and providing copies of this ruling" (USDA- FSIS, 2001). This same ruling specifies that "The constituent fax list consists of industry, trade, and farm groups, consumer interest groups, allied health professionals, scientific professionals, and other individuals who request it (USDA- FSIS, 2001).

"The reasons the food industry uses meat glue enzymes is because restructured meat can be made from underutilized portions of the carcasses. For example, the food industry can get away with adding up to 5% tendons to beef, which some people can't tell the difference. This raises food safety concerns because there is a "risk that otherwise discarded leftovers of questionable microbial quality could find its way into the reconstituted meat. If E. coli O157: H7 gets into the glue lines where meat pieces were enzymatically attached, the restructuring process can translocate fecal matter surface contamination into the interior of the meat," (Gregor M. , 2015)

"People who have problems with gluten may develop problems when ingesting meat and dairy products treated with the meat glue enzyme since it functions as an auto-antigen capable of inducing an autoimmune reaction. Many gluten-like reactions may not be due to gluten sensitivity" (Gregor M. , 2015), but rather an auto-immune response triggered by transglutaminase.

TG may trigger symptoms in people with Celiac Disease and those sensitive to gluten (Lerner, 2015).

"However, deregulation of enzyme activity generally associated with major disruptions in cellular homeostatic mechanisms has resulted in these enzymes contributing to several human diseases, including chronic neuro-degeneration, neoplastic diseases, autoimmune diseases, diseases involving progressive tissue fibrosis and diseases related to the epidermis of the skin" (Griffin, 2002).

USDA & FDA Approved:

"When transglutaminase enzyme is used to bind pieces of meat to form a cut of meat, or to reform a piece of meat from multiple cuts, there shall appear on the label, as part of the product name a statement that indicates that the product has been ``formed" or ``reformed," in addition to other preparation steps, e.g., ``Formed Beef Tenderloin" or ``Reformed and Shaped Beef Tenderloin'," (USDA- FSIS, 2001).

"Products formed from pieces of whole muscle meat, or reformed from single cuts, must disclose this fact on their label, as part of the product name, e.g., "Formed Beef Tenderloin" or "Formed Turkey Thigh Roast." The enzyme must also be listed on the product ingredient statement along with any other ingredients used in the product formulation. TG enzyme is not considered a processing aid that would be exempt from labeling. There are no exemptions to the USDA's mandatory labeling requirement for this product" (USDA-FSIS, 2017).

USDA determined that meat products sold in the supermarket that are glued together with transglutaminase are GRAS and only need to state, "formed" or "reformed" on the package (HSI, 2019).

Banned in one or more other countries: Yes

Potential Side Effects:

Allergies	Food poisoning
Auto-immune disorders	Hypertension
Cataracts	Neurological disorders
Celiac Disease	Neuro-inflammation
Cancer tumors	Skin disorders
Fibrosis	Vascular stiffness /poor circulation

TG may be bad for / Potentially aggravate and increase symptoms of the following diseases, (Robinson, 2017), (Hong, 2018), (Liu, 2017):

✓ Fatal genetic disorders that breakdown nerve cells in the

brain
- ✓ Alzheimer's disease
- ✓ Cancer
- ✓ Cardiovascular heart disease / atherosclerosis
- ✓ Cataracts
- ✓ Circulation problems
- ✓ Huntington's disease
- ✓ Hypertension
- ✓ Irritable Bowel Syndrome
- ✓ Nervous system disordered
- ✓ Ocular circulation difficulties
- ✓ Parkinson's disease

Rebekah S. Mead

References

Arnold, D. (n.d.). *Transglutaminase (Meat Glue)*. Retrieved from Molecularrecipes.com: http://www.molecularrecipes.com/hydrocolloid-guide/transglutaminase-meat-glue/

Curejoy. (2017). *What you must know about meat glue, A.K.A Transglutaminase*. Retrieved from Curejoy editorial: https://www.curejoy.com/content/what-you-must-know-about-meat-glue/

Gregor, M. (2014). *Is meat glue safe?* Retrieved from Nutrifacts.org: https://nutritionfacts.org/video/is-meat-glue-safe/

Gregor, M. (2015). What is 'Meat Glue.' *NutritionFacts.org*, https://nutritionfacts.org/2015/04/16/what-is-meat-glue/.

Hong, G. C. (2018). Inflammatory mediators resulting from transglutaminase 2 expressed in mast cells contribute to the development of Parkinson's disease in a mouse model. *Toxicology and Applied Pharmacology, 358,* 10 - 22.

Kieliszek, M. M. (2014). Microbial transglutaminase and its application in the food industry. A review. *Folia Microbiologica, 59(3),* 241-250.

Lerner, T. M. (2015). Possible association between celiac disease and bacterial transglutaminase in food processing: a hypothesis. *Nutrition Review, 73(8),* 544 - 552. Retrieved from Nutrition Review.

Liu, C. K. (2017). Inflammation, Autoimmunity, and Hypertension: The Essential Role of Tissue Transglutaminase. *American Journal of Hypertension, 30(8),* 756 - 764.

P. K. (2018). *Meat glue: What is it? What should you know?* Retrieved from Delishably: https://delishably.com/food-industry/Meat-Glue-What-It-Is-And-What-You-Should-Know

Robinson, J. (2017). *Transglutaminase — toxicity, side effects, diseases, and environmental impacts*. Retrieved from Naturalpedia: https://www.naturalpedia.com/transglutaminase-toxicity-side-effects-diseases-and-environmental-impacts.html

Romeih, E. W. (2017). Recent advances in microbial transglutaminase and dairy application. *Trends in Food Science & Technology, v.62,* 133-140.

Torsten, L. A. (2018). Microbial Transglutaminase Is Immunogenic and potentially pathogenic in pediatric celiac disease. *Frontiers in Pediatrics, 6,* 389.

USDA- FSIS. (2001). *Use of Transglutaminase Enzyme and Pork Collagen as Binders in.* Retrieved from United States Department of Agriculture - Food Safety Inspection Services: https://www.fsis.usda.gov/OPPDE/rdad/FRPubs/01-016DF.htm?redirecthttp=true

USDA-FSIS. (2017). *Safety of Transglutaminase Enzyme (TG enzyme).* Retrieved from USDA-FSIS: https://www.fsis.usda.gov/wps/portal/fsis/topics/food-safety-education/get-answers/food-safety-fact-sheets/food-labeling/safety-of-transglutaminase-tg-enzyme/safety-of-tg-enzyme

Trisodium Phosphate

Alternate names, (a.k.a.): TSP, TKP, E339, E340, tribasic calcium phosphate, tribasic calcium phosphate

Purpose: Enhance flavor, thickening agent, prevent caking, buffer. It is used to change the acidity in foods such as cereals. It is added to raw seafood, poultry, meat, and deli meats to improve tenderness.

Found in: Cheese, cereals, cereal bars, canned soups, graham crackers, pizza dough, soda, diet beverages, toothpaste, baby toothpaste, mouthwash, and processed meats. Acts as a leavening agent in many commercial cakes and baked goods. Also found in some pet foods.

Daily Recommended Amount: Maximum of 70 mg per day

"However, it is consumed as part of a Western junk food diet, and some people intake over 500mg per day, leading to numerous adverse events (HealthGuide.net, 2018).

Nutritional Value: "Phosphorus, like nitrogen, is a critical nutrient required for all life. The most common form of phosphorus used by biological organisms is phosphate (PO_4), which plays major roles in the formation of DNA, cellular energy, and cell membranes (and plant cell walls). Phosphorus is a common ingredient in commercial fertilizers," "However, in excess quantities, phosphorus can lead to water quality problems, (EPA, 2019).

Additional Information:

Potassium is an electrolyte; Trisodium phosphate is a buffer that can cause changes in our potassium balance. This can have an adverse effect heart, kidney, and digestive system functions such as peristalsis.

"Food-grade trisodium phosphate is much-diluted, purified, and used in small amounts in food. It is not the technical-grade chemical found in paint thinner and many other products.

However, one concern about phosphate additives, in general, is that they are very well absorbed—sometimes up to 100 percent—which can lead to elevated blood levels. In contrast, only 10 to 60 percent often naturally occurring phosphates widely found in meat, poultry, seafood, dairy foods, nuts, seeds, beans, and whole grains are absorbed. And elevated blood levels have been linked in some (though not all) studies to a spectrum of health problems, notably cardiovascular events—not just in people with kidney disease, who have long been advised to limit their phosphorus intake, including phosphate additives, but also in healthy people. It's thought that phosphates may damage blood vessels, impair endothelial function (which allows blood vessels to dilate), and promote calcification in blood vessels, all of which are linked to atherosclerosis, (Larsson, 2010)

For instance, a 2010 study found an association between blood phosphorus levels and cardiovascular disease and death, including in people with no heart disease at baseline (Larsson, 2010). And a 2007 study found that high blood phosphorus levels predicted cardiovascular disease (Dhingra, 2007). Other studies have linked phosphates with stiff arteries, a thickening of the wall of the carotid artery (a major artery going to the brain), and an increased risk of heart failure.

The Center for Science in the Public Interest, a D.C.-based nonprofit consumer advocacy group, advises to "cut back" on phosphates. Limiting processed foods, sodas, and "fast foods" is a sure way to reduce them in your diet. Following a predominantly whole-foods, plant-based diet, that is limited in processed foods, is also the most healthful way to eat for many other reasons. If you have chronic kidney disease, it's particularly important to watch your intake" (Barrone, 2018).

Side Effects

Allergies	Hardening of arteries
Bad breath	Hives
Bloating	Inflammation
Cancer	Irritable Bowel Syndrome
Chest pain	Muscle weakness
Confusion	Nausea
Dehydration	Respiratory distress
Diarrhea	Shock; circulatory collapse
Dizziness	Shortness of breath
Erosion of stomach lining	Stomach pains
Gassiness	Swelling, tingling lips & tongue
Glucose Intolerance	Weak pulse

Anyone taking medications to treat symptoms listed above or have the following conditions may want to avoid this additive:

- ✓ Anxiety, depression
- ✓ Colon cancer
- ✓ Dementia
- ✓ Heart disease / vascular disease
- ✓ Irritable Bowel Syndrome
- ✓ Kidney cancer/failure
- ✓ Learning disabilities
- ✓ Liver failure, fatty liver, cancer
- ✓ Mood disorders
- ✓ Stomach ulcers

References

Barrone, J. (2018). *Istrisodium phosphate in our food really paint thinner?* Retrieved from Berkley Wellness; University of Berkley: https://www.berkeleywellness.com/healthy-eating/food-safety/article/trisodium-phosphate-food-really-paint-thinner

Dhingra, R. S. (2007). Relations of serum phosphorus and calcium levels to the incidence of cardiovascular disease in the community. *Arch Intern, Med., 167(9)*, 879-885.

EPA. (2019). *Indicators: Phosphorus.* Retrieved from Environmental Protection Agency: https://www.epa.gov/national-aquatic-resource-surveys/indicators-phosphorus

HealthGuide.net. (2018). *Tripotassium phosphate vs. trisodium phosphate In cereals – Dangers and uses.* Retrieved from Health guide: https://healthguidenet.com/foods/tripotassium-phosphate-vs-trisodium-phosphate/

Larsson, T. O. (2010). Larsson TE1, Olauson H, Hagström E, Ingelsson E, Arnlöv J, Lind L, Sundström J. *Arterioscler Thromb Vasc Biol., 30(2),* 333-339.

Abbreviations

Abbreviation	Definition
a.k.a.	alternate names used for the same food additive
ADHD	Attention Deficit Hyperactivity Disorder
ADI	Acceptable Daily Intake
AHA	American Heart Association
AMS	Agriculture Marketing System
ANA	American Nutrition Association
APM	Aspartame
Cgn	Carrageenan
CPFBSs	Cartagena Protocols for Biotechnology Standards of Safety
DNA	Deoxyribonucleic Acid
EBR	Evidence-Based Research
e-coli	Escherichia-coli
EO	Executive Orders
EPA	Environmental Protection Act
FDA	Food and Drug Administration
FRM	Food Reference Manual
FSIS	Food Safety Inspection Services
GE	Genetically engineered
GI	Gastrointestinal tract or system
Gm	grams
GMO	Genetically Modified Organisms
GRAS	Generally Recognized as Safe.
GSHC	FDA term for "Generally Safe for Human Consumption
GURT	Genetic Use of Restrictive Technologies
HDL	High-Density Lipoproteins
HFCS	High fructose corn syrup
HGT	Horizontal Gene Transfer

HT	Herbicide Tolerant
IARC	International Agency for Research on Cancer
IFPS	International Federation for Produce Standards
IFPS	The International Federation for Produce Standards
LDL	Low-Density Lipoproteins
mg	milligrams
ml	milliliters
MSDS	Material Safety Data Sheet
MSG	Mono Sodium Glutamate
n.d.	No date
NLEA	Nutrition Labeling and Education Act
OFPA	Organic Foods Production Act of 1990
OTC	Over the Counter
PDP	Pesticide Data Program
PLU	Product Look Up code
POB	Products of Biotechnology
RCA	Root Cause Analysis
RISC	THE REGULATORY Information Service Center
SCFA	Short Chain Fatty Acids
SDS (MSDS)	Safety Diagnostic Standards
TC	Total Cholesterol
TC / HD	Total Cholesterol divided by High Density
TG enzymes	Transglutaminase enzymes
USDA	United States Department of Agriculture
VGT	Vertical Gene Transfer
VLDL	Very Low-Density Lipoproteins
WHO	World Health Organization

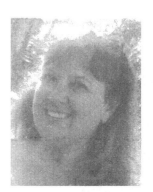

Meet the Author

Rebekah Sue Mead RN, BSN, MSN Ed., FND, HWC, believes in the spirit of environmental health and safety nursing with a focus on public health awareness. Her associate degree in nursing was earned in 1986 from the Raritan Valley Community College. The instructors and nursing curriculum at that time strongly accentuated holistic nursing care with an emphasis on Dorothea Orem's theory of nursing. Being a natural historian, Rebekah also revered Florence Nightingale's foundation of modern nursing.

As a child, Rebekah loved gardening, cooking, and creative writing. Her mother was a Mennonite, raised in Lancaster, Pennsylvania. She left the community to attend college in 1927 -1932. It was Rebekah's mother's deep-rooted belief in natural health that predisposed Rebekah to holistic health, hard work, and healthy eating. This prompted her interest in understanding the cause of illness as well as providing treatment. It was the articles by Florence Nightingale that supported her belief that fresh (unpolluted) air, exercise, and clean food are the basis of good health and quality of life.

In Philadelphia Pa and Elizabeth NJ, Rebekah was first a bedside nurse, mostly caring for patients with AIDs, which were specialty units back then. She then became an intensive care nurse specializing in head and spinal cord injuries. In 2004, Rebekah became the Executive Director of the Catskill Rural Aids Services. It was during this time that she wrote articles and produced a monthly newsletter for clients affected and infected with HIV. She was a frequent guest on two local radio stations and was interviewed three times by the channel 2 news.

Rebekah also has a Forensic Nurse Diploma (FND). This opened the door to be a Sexual Assault Nurse at Lehigh Valley Medical Center, and case-management of workers compensation insurance claims for multiple insurance companies. Rebekah earned her bachelor's and masters' degrees from the Thomas Edison State College of NJ. During this time, her electives included the biology of nutrition. Rebekah's master's degree is in Nursing Education. After graduating from TESC, Rebekah worked as an occupational health and safety nurse. This experience brought together all of her experience and education in environmental health.

Now living in Florida, Rebekah has an organic garden, loves to cook, and is back to writing. Rebekah has begun a new chapter in her life with her first book, What's Eating You? A Food Reference Manual.

Rebekah S. Mead

Made in the USA
Lexington, KY
07 December 2019